T0197209

HOW TO GET
PREGNANT
NATURALLY

JUDY McKAY

BALBOA.PRESS
A DIVISION OF HAY HOUSE

Balboa Press books may be ordered through booksellers or by contacting:

Balboa Press
A Division of Hay House
1663 Liberty Drive
Bloomington, IN 47403
www.balboapress.com
1 (877) 407-4847

Because of the dynamic nature of the Internet, any web addresses or links contained in
this book may have changed since publication and may no longer be valid. The views
expressed in this work are solely those of the author and do not necessarily reflect the
views of the publisher, and the publisher hereby disclaims any responsibility for them.

The author of this book does not dispense medical advice or prescribe the use of any
technique as a form of treatment for physical, emotional, or medical problems without the
advice of a physician, either directly or indirectly. The intent of the author is only to offer
information of a general nature to help you in your quest for emotional and spiritual well-
being. In the event you use any of the information in this book for yourself, which is your
constitutional right, the author and the publisher assume no responsibility for your actions.

The information, ideas, and suggestions in this book are not intended as a substitute
for professional medical advice. Before following any suggestions contained in
this book, you should consult your personal physician. Neither the author nor the
publisher shall be liable or responsible for any loss or damage allegedly arising as a
consequence of your use or application of any information or suggestions in this book.

Any people depicted in stock imagery provided by Getty Images are models,
and such images are being used for illustrative purposes only.
Certain stock imagery © Getty Images.

Print information available on the last page.

ISBN: 978-1-9822-4681-5 (sc)
ISBN: 978-1-9822-4683-9 (hc)
ISBN: 978-1-9822-4682-2 (e)

Library of Congress Control Number: 2020907583

Balboa Press rev. date: 07/20/2020

Contents

Contents

Introduction

My journey to getting pregnant naturally officially began when I was involved in a car accident while working in Hawaii in August 1994. I was in a parking lot, and somebody backed into my car. After the accident, my neck was stiff, so I found a local chiropractor. She was a very cheerful person and radiated positive energy. After each treatment, I felt better physically and mentally. After several weeks, she recommended that I undergo polarity therapy and massage. I was very fortunate to get one of the top masseurs in Hawaii. She was excellent. We were talking about the accident, and she told me she believed there was no such thing as an accident. She said things happen for a reason, and although we don't know why at the time, we usually find out later. I told her during the course of my treatment that I was trying to get pregnant (I told everyone I met). She told me to contact her when I got pregnant. She suggested I try acupuncture when I got home.

I went to the acupuncturist in October 1994. She recommended that I see a Chinese doctor. The doctor prescribed a variety of herbs to balance my body. While at the office, I saw a brochure for Chi Nei Tsang and the six healing sounds. It looked interesting, so I decided to try it. I felt like I was embarking on a journey that would result in me getting pregnant. I was excited to know that I would learn many new things about my body in the process. The practitioner who performed Chi Nei Tsang taught me about

Chinese medicine and how the Chinese believe that different organs carry your emotions. She taught me how to do the inner smile and the six healing sounds. She told me to avoid cold foods. Her methods were very different, but I desperately wanted to get pregnant, so I followed her directions. She was also going to the same Chinese doctor. I even convinced my husband to go to her too.

She also recommended a therapist who also did bodywork. The therapist said my heart was closed, and it needed to be open to conceive a child. I was concentrating on getting pregnant and was under so much stress, so my husband and I decided to take a break. I focused on improving myself and did not think about getting pregnant. I signed up for a yoga class in September 1995 and started meditating. I also joined an infertility support group through RESOLVE.

I continued seeing the Chinese doctor and taking the herbs he prescribed, but the prescriptions were in Chinese, so I had no idea what I was taking. So I did my own research. While looking at a local alternative medicine magazine, I saw a class on herbs that taught treatments and remedies for the systems of the body. I signed up for a class on the female reproductive system. The treatments included herbs for endometriosis and fibroid tumors (both of which I had). The class began in September 1995. The herbalist recommended herbs for both conditions, so I began drinking herb tea daily. The herbs smelled terrible! It was so bad that my husband made me brew the tea outside. He thought I had gone crazy. I told him it was cheaper than fertility drugs and in vitro fertilization.

In the middle of November 1995, at thirty-six years old, much to my surprise, I became pregnant! We did three home pregnancy tests because we didn't believe it. In August 1996, we became the proud parents of a beautiful, healthy baby girl! Our dream finally came true after a long and trying four and a half years.

We started trying for a second child when my daughter was a year old. I had a feeling that I was still on a journey and I needed to go another route. I had a strong feeling that the herbs would not work for me, so I meditated and trusted my intuition to find the right method this time. Through reading the book *Friendship with God* by Neale Donald Walsch, I learned about Dahnhak / Body and Brain. Dahnhak is a Korean mind/body training program that teaches how to develop your mind and body by enabling you to feel and utilize the ki energy. I began going to classes in March 2000, and by the end of April, I was pregnant again at age forty. I had another healthy baby girl in January 2001, at the age of forty-one.

In this book, I will introduce you to the various paths I took to become pregnant. We discussed going the conventional method (i.e., fertility drugs and in vitro fertilization) but decided against it because the success rate was low, and it was very expensive. In addition, I was not comfortable with the long-term effects of the fertility drugs on my body. Prior to 1994, I had four laparoscopies. During two of the four laparoscopies, they did laser surgery to remove endometriosis. I also had uterine fibroids. The only conventional drug I used was Clomid and Inter Uterine Insemination (IUI) for four months. I also monitored my temperature and cervical mucus daily during that time.

Everything presented in this book, I have personally experienced. Chapter 1 presents the sobering facts on infertility by traditional methods. It is much more common than you would think.

Chapter 2 will cover the topic of Chinese medicine. The Chinese believe that we are connected with nature, heaven, and earth. This includes the principles of yin and yang and how qi flows in our bodies. I will explain the five elements—wood, fire, earth, metal, and water—and how they affect our energy. I will present some easy and quick "sexercises" designed to increase sexual energy for both men and women. This chapter also includes a discussion of acupuncture, suggested herbs and vitamins designed to increase fertility, and easy Chi Nei Tsang practices, including the six healing sounds for your organs and the inner smile to balance and relax the body.

Chapter 3 outlines how Reiki energy healing techniques affect the chakras. It explains what each chakra does and how emotions affect them.

Chapter 4 includes a mind/body method, Dahnhak / Body and Brain, that I used to become pregnant with my second child. This is a combination of yoga, exercises, meditation and breathing techniques.

Chapter 5 covers some mind/body methods to achieve pregnancy, including massage, relaxation techniques, meditation, imagery/visualization, polarity therapy, and yoga.

Chapter 6 explains another powerful Chinese healing method, Qi Gong, and how it can be used to relax your body to help you get pregnant.

Chapter 7 covers nutrition and suggested foods to eat to clean and balance your body so you can be in optimal shape to get pregnant.

Chapter 8 provides other information that could also help, including support groups, chiropractic information, emotional freedom technique (EFT), and general information I found during my research. I will also mention other methods that I didn't use to get pregnant but that I have used after having my children and that have helped other women get pregnant.

I believe the mind plays a very important part in getting pregnant. Before my first pregnancy, we had attended a seminar on adopting a baby girl from China. We had drafted up a letter to the adoption agency when I found out I was pregnant. We were looking into adopting a boy when I got pregnant again. I believe once I made up my mind that a child was what I really wanted, then my body cooperated. I was also going to an infertility support group.

If you try one of the methods in this book and it doesn't work for you, don't give up! Try another one. Every woman's body is different, and depending on your issues, you might need to try different methods. What worked for me the first time didn't work the second time. It is easy to get discouraged but ask for guidance from the higher power, and you will get it.

If everything worked out like I had planned, I would have had my children in my early thirties when we started trying. But I had my children at ages thirty-six and forty-one. I believe God has a plan for us, and we have to be open to whatever life gives us. I guess God wanted me to embark on this journey before I became a mother. I learned so much in the process! My father was forty-five when I was born, and my husband was forty-five when my second daughter was born. Coincidence? I think not.

This book took me more than ten years to write. I believe it took so long because along the way, I learned about other methods that would help you get pregnant. All of these methods are included, and even though I didn't use all of them to get pregnant, I know other women who became pregnant using them.

The road to getting pregnant has been a strange and wonderful journey. During the process, I learned so much about alternative medicine, my body, and myself. Because this journey took me in so many directions, I wanted to share my story and what I have learned about natural ways to get pregnant. If you have tried conventional methods with no success, or just want to learn about alternative (and much cheaper) methods to achieving pregnancy, then you owe it to yourself to read this. After all, having a child is your dream. Children are truly gifts from God! They are definitely worth the wait. So, open your mind and heart to new possibilities and learn everything you can about natural ways to get pregnant.

Chapter 1

Infertility Facts

Infertility is all too common these days. The diagnosis of infertility is usually given to couples who have been attempting to conceive for at least one year, and for women over thirty-five, at least six months without success. The statistics are sobering. According to the National Survey of Family Growth in the Center for Disease Control and Prevention, 6.7 million women in the United States are unable to have a child. This affects one in every nine women in the United States—about 11 percent of the reproductive age population. Infertility affects men and women equally. Twenty-five percent of infertile couples have more than one factor contributing to their infertility. Most infertility cases (85–90 percent) are treated with conventional medical therapies such as medication or surgery.[1]

The most common assisted reproductive technology (ART) is in vitro fertilization, or IVF. Other ARTs include GIFT (gamete intrafallopian transfer) and ZIFT (zygote intrafallopian transfer).[2] Fertility medications are required prior to the procedures. However, there are many side effects and risks from these procedures, and the success rates range from only 13 to 43 percent. Some of the side effects of IVF include cramping, bloating, constipation, breast tenderness, and passing fluid after the procedure. More serious side effects include heavy vaginal bleeding, pelvic pain, blood in the urine, and a fever over 100.5°F. Side effects of fertility medications may include headaches, mood swings, abdominal pain, hot flashes, abdominal bloating, and sometimes ovarian hyperstimulation syndrome. More severe symptoms include nausea, decreased urinary frequency, shortness of breath, faintness, severe stomach pains and bloating, and ten-pound weight gain within three to five days. Additional risks of IVF include risks of bleeding, infection and damage to the bowel or bladder, chance of multiple pregnancies, psychological stress and emotional problems if unsuccessful, and ectopic pregnancy.[3]

It is also very expensive. The average cost for a single IVF cycle in the United States can range from $12,000 to $17,000.[4] The cost is usually not covered by insurance; however, fifteen states currently cover a portion of infertility diagnosis and treatment.[3]

The success rate of IVF clinics depends on reproductive history, maternal age, the cause of infertility, and lifestyle factors. In the United States, the live birth rate for each IVF cycle started is approximately:

- 41–43 percent for women under thirty-five
- 33–36 percent for women thirty-five to thirty-seven
- 23–27 percent for women thirty-eight to thirty-nine
- 13–18 percent for women over forty[4]

So, for women under thirty-five, less than 44 percent had success! Those odds weren't good enough for me. I knew several people who had done IVF without success. My husband and I discussed going the traditional route, but because of the high cost, low success rate, and the unknown long-term effects of the fertility medicines, we opted to look at alternate ways to get pregnant. I wanted children, but I didn't want to risk getting cancer or having some other problems later in life.

According to the American Fertility Association, any medication that causes unusual hormone production could potentially cause cancer in the reproductive system. Some fertility drugs, such as clomiphene, can actually induce additional fertility complications in some women, according to the American Fertility Association. Clomiphene, commonly marketed as Clomid, forces ovulation. But the drug can cause the lining of the uterus not to be adequately prepared to hold an embryo and sometimes also creates an environment within the body that can see sperm as hostile and not permit fertilization.[5] Common side effects include ovarian cysts and enlargement of the ovaries. Some of the rare, but more serious side effects of Clomiphene include: breast cancer, cancer of the lining of the uterus, endometriosis, thinning of the uterine lining, and ovarian hyperstimulation syndrome - an abnormal enlargement of the ovaries and tumors.[6]

A study published in the *Canadian Medical Association Journal* (CMAJ) examined years of health data on women who received fertility treatment in Ontario. It found women who received fertility treatment but did not give birth were 19 percent more likely to experience a cardiovascular event, particularly heart failure, compared with those who gave birth within one year of fertility treatment.[7]

The study, funded by the Heart and Stroke Foundation of Canada and the Canada Research Chair in Medical Decision Science, analyzed data on 28,442 women, fifty and younger, who received fertility therapy in Ontario between 1993 and 2011. Of these, 33 percent gave birth within one year after receiving their last fertility treatment, while 67 percent did not. The median number of fertility treatments was three. Researchers found 2,686 cardiovascular events occurred over a median 8.4 years after receiving treatment.[7]

Dr. Jacob Udell, lead author of the study, a scientist at the Institute for Clinical Evaluative Sciences and a cardiologist at the Peter Munk Cardiac Centre at Toronto General Hospital and Women's

College Hospital, suggested there are two possible explanations for the increased risk of heart disease and stroke found in women for whom fertility therapy failed. The first is that fertility treatment may act as a metabolic stress test; when it is unsuccessful, it unmasks or points out individuals who may have medical problems later in life. The other possibility is that exposure to fertility drugs could lead to a higher risk of heart failure and stroke.[7]

I chose Chinese medicine with its many forms of energy healing because it made perfect sense to me to go the natural route and not take the risks associated with getting pregnant by artificial means.

Chapter 2

Chinese Medicine

The road I took to get pregnant primarily involved Chinese medicine. The Chinese have it right. Their medical system began almost three thousand years ago and is based on a belief that we are connected with nature and heaven and earth. The connection among heaven, earth, and each human being is a living energy, called the life force or qi. The Chinese believe that heaven and earth combine to create qi, which flows through humans, maintaining our health and leading us to our destiny. Whereas Western medicine treats the symptoms individually, the Chinese treat the whole body as one system.[8]

The Chinese believe that all illness arises from imbalance, or a condition where there is excess in someone's life: weakness, strength, wealth, poverty, food or drink, or a particular way of thinking. The goal of Chinese medicine is to restore a person's health, balance, and harmony on all levels—physical, mental, emotional, and spiritual—by helping to stimulate the body's own self-healing powers.[8]

The yin and the yang represent opposite forces in nature. The yin represents things when they contract or are passive, cool, wet, and slow-moving. Yin is the female principle. The earth and the moon are yin. Things in a relaxed state are yin. Yang represents things when they expand, become active, fiery, hot, dry, and fast-moving. Yang is the masculine principle. Heaven and the sun are yang. Stressful conditions are considered yang. When the yin and yang in the body are disturbed and either one becomes excessive, disease or emotional problems can result.[9]

Yin and yang cause the movement of qi, but each of us is responsible for maintaining the flow of the life force within our physical bodies. Our behavior determines the degree to which the life force flows through us, whether we expand the life force or engage in behaviors that diminish the flow of qi within us.[9]

We control the qi in the body by our thinking, daily activity, diet, exercise habits, and our emotional condition. One of the primary tools Chinese healers use to boost qi flow is acupuncture (see Page 13). The Chinese believe that if qi flow is restored, health can also be restored. Therefore, healers treat disease by increasing the flow of qi to the diseased part of the body. They focus their healing on certain organs and tissues that may have deficient or excessive qi and try to bring these organs into balance.[9]

The Chinese believe that energy moves throughout the body in a precise pattern,. They use the five elements, or phases (wood, fire, earth, metal, and water), to understand and chart how the qi moves through the body. They represent five different movements of energy, energetic tendencies, and vibratory rates.[10] Wood represents the spring, budding growth, and expansion. The organs are the liver (primary) and the gallbladder (secondary). Fire represents accomplishment and abundance. The heart is the primary organ for fire, and the small intestine is the secondary organ. Earth represents balance and neutrality. The organs that represent earth are the stomach (primary) and spleen (secondary). Metal represents contraction and condensation. The corresponding organs are the lungs (primary) and large intestine (secondary). The last phase element is water, which represents fall, a time of rest, darkness, and stillness. The organs that represent water are the kidneys (primary) and the bladder (secondary).[11]

The Chinese believe water is the foundation, root, and source of life, so the reproductive system is governed by this phase. So, if the kidney energy is not functioning properly, this could affect the reproductive system. The time of day that the bladder receives the most abundant energy is from 3:00 p.m. to 5:00 p.m., and the kidneys are from 5:00 p.m. to 7:00 p.m. Most practitioners of acupuncture and Chinese herbal treatment feel confident they can improve fertility in women.[12]

In Chinese medicine, the sexual vitality of men and women depends on the health of the kidneys and adrenal glands, which are located on top of the kidneys. Infertility is due to kidney yang deficiency, meaning the absence of warmth and outgoing energy (fire energy). They even suggest wearing a cotton cummerbund around the kidneys, adrenals, and bladder beneath your shirt to keep the kidneys warm.[13] That is why my practitioner told me to eat warm or hot foods and stay away from cold foods when I was trying to get pregnant.

According to *The Complete Book of Chinese Health and Healing* by Daniel Reid, the Chinese also practice certain chee-gung exercises to enhance sexual energy. They are designed to directly stimulate the testicles and ovaries (also known as the outer kidneys) by inducing the testicles, ovaries, and other sexual glands to secrete elevated levels of hormones.[14] (See pages 8 to 13.)

The Chinese believe the energy derived from hormones is stored primarily in the two reservoirs formed by the leg vessels of the eight extraordinary channels. When this energy is drawn upward from the legs into the central and governor channels by deep breathing, visualization, chee-gung, and meditation, the extra sexual essence produced by the sexercises is converted into energy and stored in the leg channels to replace the energy that has been drawn up from those channels into the higher energy centers.[15]

The Governor Channel runs from the perineum, up the spine, to the head. At the head, it enters the brain, runs over the crown, down to the midpoint between the eyes, and ends at the roof of the mouth, where it connects with the Functional Channel. The Governor Channel is closely associated with the brain, spinal fluid, and the reproductive system.[16]

As sexual energy is drawn up from the leg channels, it is further refined as it rises upward through the energy centers into the brain, where it is transformed into pure spiritual vitality. As it rises, it cleanses and energizes the marrow, fluids, and nerves of the spine.[15]

Sexercises may be practiced any time of the day or night. You should prepare your body and energy channels with a few stretches and some deep breathing and finish with ten or fifteen minutes of standing still or sitting to harvest your enhanced sexual energy and move it into general circulation through your channels for storage in the lower abdomen. You should never leave hot sexual energy floating in your brain after practicing solo sexercises, or you will have headaches and dizziness.[15]

For Women and Men

Pelvic Thrust

Technique: Stand in horse stance, with the feet pointed forward, thighs parallel to the floor, with the buttocks pushed out, and the back arched up to keep the upper body from leaning forward. Place hands on hips and slightly bend the knees. Inhale and slowly thrust the pelvis back as far as possible, arching the lower spine and sticking the butt out. Then exhale and draw the pelvis forward, straightening the lower spine and tucking the butt in as far as possible. Continue this for two or three minutes. You may also use this as a warm-up exercise.[17]

Benefits: Stimulates and stretches the nerve fibers in the sacral region, thereby stimulating secretions of sexual energy in testicles, ovaries, prostate, and other sacral glands. Limbers and tones the vertebrae and nerves of the lower spine, which regulate sexual functions. Stimulates kidney and bladder organ energies. Draws blood and energy into the sacrum, enhancing sexual energy. Encourages energy to rise up from the leg channels to the perineum, where it enters circulation in the energy channels. This triggers conversion of sexual essence into sexual energy to replace the energy drawn up from the legs.[17]

Embracing Tree in wide stance on toes

Technique: Adopt a wide stance, with feet turned outward at a forty-five-degree angle. Raise arms into embracing tree posture, with fingertips of hands aligned, thumbs up, and hands held at throat level. Tuck in the butt, straighten up the back of the neck, and stand up on the toes and balls of the feet. Breathe slowly and deeply, focusing your attention on the fingertips and bones of the hands and keeping the anal sphincter slightly contracted to prevent energy from escaping. On inhalation, imagine energy entering in a spiral through the fingertips and spinning up through the bones of the hands into the arms, then down the chest into the lower abdomen, where it accumulates. Then exhale and visualize energy spiraling up the spine from the lower abdomen to the head. This is a good exercise for practicing reverse abdominal breathing, which intensifies the effects.[18]

At first, you won't be able to hold this posture very long, but as the muscles, tendons, and energy in your legs build up, you'll be able to practice it for increasingly longer periods. Try starting with four to six deep abdominal breaths and work up to a dozen or more.[18]

Benefits: This exercise builds up the muscles and tendons attaching the thighs to the hips and pelvis and draws energy up from the legs and down from the arms and chest into the sacral region, where it stimulates sexual secretions. It strengthens the sexual organs in men and women, builds up the lumbar vertebrae (which regulate sexual functions), and encourages energy to rise up from the leg channels and enter the upper channels via the perineum.[19]

Jade Hop

Technique: This exercise should be performed naked. Place your feet a bit wider than shoulder width apart and parallel to each other. Raise your arms above the head, with elbows bent, shoulders relaxed and palms facing each other. Straighten up the back of the neck, slightly contract the anus, and start hopping gently up and down at a fairly brisk pace. As you hop, slowly curl the fingers into fists and relax them, repeating rhythmically but at a slower pace than the hopping. For men, the hopping should cause the penis to flap up and down, slapping against the stomach above the perineum below, while the testicles bounce up and down. For women, the hopping should cause the breasts to bounce up and down. Continue until you feel winded, which will only take two or three minutes at first. Eventually you'll be able to continue for longer periods.[19]

Benefits: For men, this exercise strongly stimulates the testicles and prostate and greatly enhances circulation of blood and energy to the penis. For women, it stimulates the ovaries and enhances circulation in the uterus and vagina. It also stimulates blood circulation and sexual secretions in women's breasts. For both men and women, hopping stimulates the pituitary gland in the brain and the thymus gland over the heart. It builds up strength and stamina in the adrenals, which play a major role in regulating sexual vitality. It also prevents formation of kidney stones by shaking up the contents of the kidneys, which helps dissolve crystals before they form.[20]

For Women Only

Ovary Massage

Technique: Stand relaxed in horse stance and warm up with a few minutes of deep breathing. Rub your palms together till warm, then place thumbs together at the navel, forming a straight line from thumb to thumb parallel to the ground. Then place the tips of the index fingers together to form a triangle. The ovaries are located at the tips of the little and ring fingers. Use those fingers to massage the ovaries in a circular mention thirty-six times in one direction, then thirty-six times in the other. Keeping the hands in this position on the abdomen, do a few minutes of deep abdominal breathing to draw warm sexual energy upward along the spine into the head, then back down the front into the lower elixir field (about two inches below the navel) for storage. Contract the anus on inhalation and relax it on exhalation in order to stimulate energy into circulation.[21]

Benefits: Increases sexual secretions from ovaries, stimulates female sexual energy, and helps regulate menstrual cycles. If you have ovarian cysts or similar problems, do this exercise two or three times daily, in order to stimulate circulation of blood and healing energy into these tissues.[21]

Nipple Massage

Technique: Stand in horse stance, or sit comfortably on a hard stool or chair, with bare feet on the floor. Close your eyes and do a few minutes of deep breathing. Then rub the palms together until warm. Then place the center of the palms firmly over your nipples and slowly massage in circles, thirty-six times in one direction and thirty-six times in the other. You may also use the tips of the index, middle, and ring fingers to massage in circles in a one-inch radius around the nipples. As you massage, focus attention on the point between the eyebrows, the throat, then the heart, the kidneys, and finally the ovaries, drawing warm sexual energy to those centers.

11

Do one to three sets. When finished, stand or sit still for a while with your eyes closed to let the energy circulate up the back and down the front.[22]

Benefits: This exercise is often prescribed for frigidity or low libido, because it stimulates female sexual energy. It also turns on the entire female endocrine system. By focusing attention on various glandular centers (pituitary in brain, thyroid in throat, thymus at heart), warm sexual energy is drawn to those points and stimulates those glands. This is also a good way for women to warm up their channels before practicing internal energy meditation.[22]

For Men Only

Dragon Pearl Testicle Massage

Technique: Stand in horse stance or sit on the edge of a hard stool or chair without pants. Rub your palms together until warm, then place the tips of all four fingers underneath the testicles, with thumbs on top, and massage the testicles firmly by rolling them around between the fingertips and thumbs. Pressure should be firm but not painful. Roll the testicles thirty-six times in each direction. Then relax and draw energy upward with abdominal breathing, performed along with anal lock and visualization.[22]

Benefits: Increases production of testosterone, sperm, and seminal fluids and elevates male sexual energy. When energy is drawn upward from the leg channels, the extra sexual essence produced by testicle massage will be converted to energy and stored in the leg channels.[23]

Dragon Tendon Seminal-Duct Massage

Technique: Hold the testicles in the same manner as above, but instead of massaging the testicles, use the tips of the ring fingers and thumbs to locate the seminal ducts above the testicles. When you've found them, roll these tubes around between the fingertips and thumbs. Then pinch and release them. Then stretch them downward like rubber bands. Be careful and gentle.[23]

Benefits: Clears the seminal ducts of stagnant seminal fluids, tones the tissues of the ducts, and stimulates sperm and semen production.[23]

Acupuncture

According to the Chinese system, Qi flows through the body in fourteen distinct patterns, called meridians. When Qi flows freely through these meridians, the body receives optimal amounts of life force.[24] Acupuncture is an energy medicine, acting on the body's energy system to change the mind and body.[25] Acupuncture is performed on the fourteen meridians all over the body. The main meridians are all connected with the organs and include the small intestine, bladder, gall bladder, triple heater, colon, stomach, lung, spleen, heart governor, liver, heart, and kidneys. There are about three hundred sixty-five acupuncture points on the body.[26]

Acupuncture treatment concentrates on the whole person, not just the disease. Acupuncture's aim is to build up the body's own powers of self-defense, instead of bringing in outside forces to help fight disease.[27] To the acupuncturist, if the spirit is not balanced, the whole system lacks control and direction. It is just as important that problems of the spirit are treated by rebalancing, removing blockages, and restoring the natural flow of energy. The Chinese do not distinguish between physical and mental problems like Western medicine; both are treated at the same time by the same doctor. Most people find acupuncture treatment relaxing.[28] After getting an acupuncture treatment, I feel like I had just had a massage. It feels wonderful! I would highly recommend it!

The acupuncturist will spend a lot of time asking questions about the patient's general condition. Although some of the questions may seem unrelated, all of them can help the acupuncturist form a complete picture of the patient's condition.

A full medical history is also taken, including past illnesses, operations, and other traumas, both mental and physical. Women will be asked about their menstrual cycle, including the length, duration and heaviness and the amount of pain they experience during menstruation. They will also take the patient's pulse on both wrists. This reading is considered to be the acupuncturist's main diagnostic tool. The pulse is taken at both wrists and in three positions, by the index, middle and ring finger. They will also ask to look at the patient's tongue. Different colors of the tongue relate to certain deficiencies in the body. Certain points on the tongue also relate to different organs.[29]

The Chinese doctor I visited took my pulse and looked at my tongue. After he did, he asked me questions about certain problems I had. It was amazing that he knew exactly what my problems were just by taking my pulse and looking at my tongue. The pulse and the tongue are the acupuncturist's most important diagnostic tools. These simple methods are very important to a person's healing.

The needles used in acupuncture are extremely fine and usually are made of stainless steel or they are disposable. The needles should not cause pain when they are inserted, but you may feel tingling when the Qi starts to flow or you may have a brief feeling of numbness initially.[30]

Cupping is another type of treatment that may be done during acupuncture. This is a method of stimulating acupuncture points by applying suction through a metal, wood, or glass jar in which a partial vacuum has been created. This technique produces blood congestion at the site and therefore stimulates it. It is used to remove stagnation. Cupping is used for low backache, sprains, soft tissue injuries, and helping relieve fluid from the lungs in chronic bronchitis.[31]

There are several organizations that you can contact for more information on acupuncture or to find an acupuncturist in your area. These include the American Association of Acupuncture and Oriental Medicine (www.AAAOMonline.org), the American Society of Acupuncturists (www.asacu.org), and the American Academy of Medical Acupuncture (www.medicalacupuncture.org and www.acupuncture.com).

Herbs

In China, acupuncture and herbalism are used together and complement each other. Trained acupuncturists spend at least two years studying herbalism. For my first pregnancy, I used herbs to get pregnant. I picked up a publication called *Pathways* in my local health food store. In the publication, I found an herbalist who was giving classes on herbs. I took a class on fertility and contraception. Once I started taking the herbs for my specific problems, I got pregnant within three months.

There are a variety of herbs that help with many female problems and could help infertility. These include chaste berry, asparagus root, false unicorn root, and Fo-Ti. The benefits of the chaste berry *(Vitex angus-castus)* have been used extensively for infertility. It is known to stimulate ovulation. This is a safe treatment with no significant side effects except occasional allergic rashes. This herb also alleviates many menstrual problems, including premenstrual syndrome. It naturally stimulates the production of progesterone and may be effective in reducing fibroid tumors. The proper dose for capsules is about 10 to 20 mg twice a day. Wild Yam regulates female hormones and keeps the reproductive organs healthy.[32]

Also, progesterone gel or cream (manufactured from Mexican yam or soybeans) may be applied to the skin. The progesterone prescribed to women by conventional physicians contains no real progesterone. It is comprised of related substances called *progestins* that can be absorbed orally. True natural progesterone cream may be more effective and cause fewer side effects than the conventional form.[33]

Asparagus root *(Asparagus officinalis)* is a restorative tonic for the female reproductive system. This old remedy is also used to treat a variety of women's reproductive and gynecological problems. It is used to treat infertility in women and impotence in men. False unicorn root regulates women's menstrual cycles. This herb is especially helpful in cases of painful or irregular menstruation. It usually has to be taken for at least three months to see results. Take two to five capsules up to three times a day. As a tincture, take one teaspoon up to three times a day. As a decoction, take one cup up to three times a day.[34]

Fo-Ti *(Polygonum multiflorum)*, known as Ho Shou Wu in China, is a good overall restorative tonic for the blood, kidneys, and liver. It may increase fertility and can be an aphrodisiac. Fo-Ti products are available as capsules, decoctions, and tinctures. Take one capsule up to three times a day. As a tincture, use one teaspoon up to three times a day. As a decoction, use two ounces two to four times a day.[34]

A beneficial herbal combination for fertility problems includes dong quai, false unicorn root, and raspberry. Make a decoction by boiling the dong quai and false unicorn roots in one and a half pints of water for ten minutes. Reduce to one pint. Add the aboveground portion of raspberry leaf, cover, and steep for another ten minutes. Use one ounce of the total herbs recommended. You should take at least three cups a day of the herbal combinations to increase fertility for three months. Add dong quai and ginger to chicken soup for an excellent female hormone tonic. Also use 100 to 500 mg of saffron unless you are pregnant.[35]

Because the Chinese believe that the health of the kidneys relates to the health of the sexual organs, burdock root is regarded as a strengthening herb for the entire urinary tract and sex organs. Burdock tea detoxifies blood, stimulates and tonifies kidneys and bladder, and eliminates waste and stagnation within the kidneys. Boil one or two tablespoons of stems, twigs, and leaves in one cup of water, steep for ten minutes, and drink two or three times per day.[36]

During the class, the teacher gave us some fertility tonics. These tonics came from the book *Herbal Healing for Women* by Rosemary Gladstar. It's called Rosemary's Fertility tonic and supports the adrenal glands:

> 4 ounces rehmanania
> 1 ounce astragalus root
> 1 ounce dong quai root
> 2 ounces false unicorn root
> 3 ounces wild yam root
> 1 ounce vitex berries

Another fertility tea that builds up estrogen and progesterone includes the following:

> 3 ounces wild yam root
> 2 ounces licorice root
> 1 ounce vitex berries
> 1 ounce false unicorn root
> .5 ounces cinnamon root
> .5 ounces ginger root

Another tonic you can take is an anti-endometriosis tonic:

> 3 ounces dandelion root
> 3 ounces wild yam root
> 2 ounces burdock root
> 2 ounces pau d'arco root
> 1 ounce vitex berries

1 ounce Oregon grape root
.5 ounces dong quai root
1 ounce cinnamon
1 ounce ginger

Here is another tonic for endometriosis:

2 ounces vitex berries
2 ounces life root
1 ounce black cohosh root
1 ounce wild yam root
1 ounce skullcap root

To prepare as a tea, mix two teaspoons herbal mix to one quart of water. Bring to a boil and simmer covered for at least twenty minutes. Drink three to four cups of tea throughout the day. You could also make a tincture. After simmering, strain the herbs through a sieve and put them in a gallon jar. Top it with alcohol (preferably vodka with 40 percent alcohol). Soak it for two weeks and shake it daily.[37]

Drink Ginseng tea or take Ginseng capsules. Ginseng is helpful for fertility problems if the infertility is related to weak reproductive organs.[37]

Another book that contains helpful information for fertility is *Herbs for the Childbearing Year* by Susun Weed. The first chapter is entitled Fertility Promoters. In addition to the herbs already mentioned above, she includes Red Clover flower, Nettle Leaves and Red Raspberry leaves as herbs which help fertility.[38]

An herbal tonic to enhance a man's fertility includes Asian or Siberian ginseng, damiana, and saw palmetto. Make a decoction by boiling the ginseng root in one and a half pints of water for ten minutes. Reduce to one pint. Add the aboveground parts of damiana and saw palmetto, cover, and steep for another ten minutes. Use one ounce of the total combined herbs recommended.[39]

Astragalus extract has been reported to stimulate sperm motility. Yohimbe also enhances sexual function in men. It may be taken in capsules or as a tincture.[40] My husband used the yohimbe tincture before our first and second children were conceived.

Yin-yang-huo (*Aceathus sagittatum*), a Chinese herb also called horny goatweed, is a male aphrodisiac and may increase sperm count and semen density.[40]

Heavy use of echinacea, ginkgo biloba and St. John's Wort may cause infertility in men.[40]

Another author states that there may be functional or energy causes for infertility. The first possibility is a "weak energy" pattern meaning that the main problem is lack of energy in the reproductive system. The medical tests may turn out fine, but there is not enough vitality in the uterus to quicken a new life. It may be due to a lack of energy overall, when you often feel tired, or to a lack of energy in the reproductive system or lower abdomen.

Herbs for this pattern include Beth root, False unicorn root, Yarrow and Licorice. Beth root and False unicorn root strengthen the pelvic area and reproductive system. Yarrow is a general tonic for the body and helps regulate periods and Licorice is an energy-mover.

The second possibility is an "excess mucus" pattern. There is too much mucus (phlegm) in the body or in the reproductive system. In the reproductive system, mucus may block the fallopian tubes, so the egg cannot pass from the ovary to the uterus, or it may affect the uterine lining and become too thick and hostile for an egg to become embedded.

Herbs for this pattern include Motherwort, Golden seal, Berberis and Balmony. Golden seal and Berberis clear mucus from the reproductive system and Balmony stimulates digestion and helps clear the uterus of stagnant energy. Motherwort opens the way for the other herbs to work.

The third possibility is a "poor energy circulation" pattern. Your energy does not circulate well, leading to irregular menstrual flow and stagnant areas. This affects the ovaries and fallopian tubes.

Herbs for this pattern include Blue cohosh, Motherwort and Catmint. Blue cohosh moves energy in the reproductive system. Motherwort helps regulate the periods and Catmint gently warms the reproductive organs.[41]

Chi Nei Tsang

The woman who educated me in Chi Nei Tsang helped me and at least ten other women become pregnant. The Taoist sages of ancient China found that humans often develop energy blockages in their internal organs, causing knots in their abdomens. These obstructions occur at the center of the body's vital functions and constrict the flow of energy. The negative emotions of fear, anger, anxiety, depression, and worry cause the most damage. Problems can also be caused by overwork, stress, accidents, surgery, drugs, toxins, bad food, and poor posture.[42]

If the internal organs are obstructed, they store unhealthy energies that can overflow into other bodily systems and result in negative emotions and sickness. These negative emotions and toxic energies create a cycle of negativity and stress. If the negative emotions can't find an outlet, they stay in the organs or move into the abdomen. The energy center of the body is located at the navel. When this energy becomes congested, it does not flow through the rest of the body.[42]

In the book *Chi Nei Tsang*, authors Mantak and Maneewan Chia explain that the ancient Taoists realized that negative emotions cause serious damage to our health and impair both physical and spiritual functions. They discovered that most problems could be healed once the underlying toxins and negative forces were released from the body. They developed the art of Chi Nei Tsang to recycle and transform negative energy that obstructs the internal organs and causes knots in the abdomen. Chi Nei Tsang clears out the toxins, bad emotions, and excessive heat or heat deficiencies that cause the organs to malfunction.[43]

They state that Chi Nei Tsang is a comprehensive approach to energizing, strengthening, and detoxifying the internal system. It clears out negative influences and is particularly useful in relieving intestinal blockages, cramps, knots, lumps, scar tissue, headaches, menstrual cramps, poor blood circulation, back pain, infertility, impotence, and other problems.[44] There are also techniques such as massage to help women with problems in the ovaries, uterus and fallopian tubes and several male problems.[45]

In the book *Taoist Ways to Transform Stress into Vitality,* author Mantak Chia explains that many years ago, the Taoist masters found in their meditation six sounds that were the correct frequencies to keep the organs in optimal condition by preventing and alleviating illness. They discovered that a healthy organ vibrates at a particular frequency. To accompany the six healing sounds, six accompanying postures were developed to activate the acupuncture meridians of the organs.[46] Watch him do the healing sounds at https://www.youtube.com/watch?v= yMHHhxwlt4.

The Six Healing Sounds

The six healing sounds include the lung sound, kidney sound, liver sound, heart sound, spleen sound, and the triple warmer sound. These sounds should be done daily in this order. Wait at least an hour after eating to do the sounds. Dress warmly enough not to be chilled. Remove your glasses and watch. All of the sounds are described in the following paragraphs.[46]

Six Healing Sounds

The first healing sound is the *lung sound*. The associated organ is the large intestine. The season is autumn. The negative emotions are sadness, grief, and sorrow. The positive emotions are righteousness, surrender, letting go, emptiness, and courage. The sound is "SSSSSSSSSS." The related parts of the body include the chest, inner arms, and thumbs. The sense is smell, the taste is pungent, and the color is white.[47]

1. Become aware of your lungs.
2. Take a deep breath and, following with your eyes, raise the arms up in front of you. When the hands are at eye level, begin to rotate the palms and bring them up above the head. Keep the elbows rounded. You should feel a stretch extending from the heels of the palms, along the forearms, over the elbows, along the upper arms, and into the shoulders. The lungs and chest will feel open, and breathing will be easier.
3. Close the jaws so that the teeth meet gently and part the lips slightly. Draw the corners of the mouth back, exhale, and allow your breath to escape through the spaces between the teeth, making the sound "SSSSSSSSSS," subvocally, slowly, and evenly in one breath.
4. As you do this, picture and feel the pleura (the sac covering the lungs) as becoming fully compressed, ejecting the excess heat, sick energy, sadness, sorrow, and grief.
5. When you have exhaled completely (without straining), rotate the palms down, close the eyes, and breathe into the lungs to strengthen them. Imagine a pure white light and quality of righteousness entering into your whole lungs. Float the arms down by gently lowering the shoulders.

Slowly lower them to your lap so that they rest there, palms up. Feel the energy exchange in the hands and palms.

6. Close the eyes, breathe normally, smile down to the lungs, be aware of the lungs, and imagine that you are still making the sound. Pay attention to any sensations you may feel. Try to feel the exchange of cool, fresh energy replacing hot energy.

7. When your breathing calms down, repeat the sequence three to six times.

8. For colds, flu, mucus, toothaches, smoking, asthma, emphysema, or depression, or if you want to increase the range of movement of the chest and inner arm or detoxify the lungs, repeat the sound nine, twelve, eighteen, twenty-four, or thirty-six times.

9. The lung sound can also help to eliminate nervousness when in front of a crowd. You can do the lung sound subvocally without the hand movements several times when you feel nervous in front of a crowd. This will help calm you down.[48]

The second healing sound is the *kidney sound*. The associated organ is the bladder. The element is water, and the season is winter. The negative emotion is fear, and the positive emotions are gentleness, alertness, and stillness. The sound is "WHOOOOOO." The parts of the body are the side of the foot, inner leg, and the chest. The sense is hearing, and the related body parts are ears and bones. The taste is salty, and the color is black or dark blue.

1. Become aware of the kidneys.

2. Place the legs together, ankles and knees touching. Take a deep breath as you bend forward and clasp one hand in the other; hook the hands around the knees and pull back on the arms. With the arms straight, feel the pull at the back where the kidneys are, look up, and tilt the head back without straining.

3. Round the lips and silently make a sound like you are blowing out a candle. At the same time, press the middle

abdomen, between the sternum and navel, toward the spine. Imagine the excess heat, the wet, sick energy, and fear being squeezed out from the membrane around the kidneys.

4. When you have exhaled completely, sit up and slowly breathe into the kidneys, imagining a bright blue energy as the quality of gentleness enters the kidneys. Separate the legs to a hip's width and rest the hands, palms up, on the thighs.

5. Close the eyes and breathe normally. Smile to the kidneys as you imagine that you are still making the sound. Pay attention to sensations. Be aware of the exchange of energy around the kidneys, hands, head, and legs.

6. When your breathing calms down, repeat three to six times.

7. For back pain, fatigue, dizziness, ringing in the ears, or detoxifying the kidneys, repeat nine to thirty-six times.[49]

The third healing sound is the *liver sound*. The associated organ is the gall bladder, and the element is wood. The season is spring. The negative emotions are anger and aggression, and the positive emotions are kindness, self-expansion, and identity. The sound is "SHHHHHHHH." The parts of the body are the inner legs, groin, diaphragm, and ribs. The senses are sight, tears, and eyes. The taste is sour, and the color is green.

1. Become aware of the liver and feel the connection between the eyes and the liver.

2. Place your arms at your sides, palms out. Take a deep breath as you slowly swing the arms up and over the head. Follow with the eyes.

3. Interlace the fingers and rotate the palms to face the ceiling. Push out at the heels of the palms and feel the stretch through the arms and into the shoulders. Bend slightly to the left, exerting a gentle pull on the liver.

4. Exhale on the sound "SHHHHHHHH" subvocally. Again, envision and feel the sac that encloses the liver compressing and expelling the excess heat and anger.
5. When you have exhaled completely, unlock the fingers, and pressing out with the heels of the palms, breathe into the liver slowly; imagine a bright green color quality of kindness entering the liver. Gently bring the arms back to the side by lowering the shoulders. Please your hands on your lap, palms up, and rest.
6. Close the eyes, breathe normally, smile down to the liver, and imagine you're still making the sound. Be aware of sensations. Sense the energy exchange.
7. Do this three to six times. For anger, red and watery eyes, or a sour or bitter taste, and to detoxify the liver, repeat nine to thirty-six times.[50]

The fourth healing sound is the *heart sound*. The associated organ is the small intestine. The element is fire, and the season is summer. The negative emotions are impatience, arrogance, hastiness, cruelty, and violence. The positive emotions are joy, honor, sincerity, creativity, enthusiasm, spirit, radiance, and light. The sound is "HAWWWWWW," and the parts of the body are the armpits and inner arms. The senses include speech and tongue. The taste is bitter, and the color is red.

1. Become aware of the heart and feel the tongue connected with the heart.
2. Take a deep breath and assume the same position as the liver sound but lean slightly to the right.
3. Open the mouth slightly, round the lips, and exhale on the sound "HAWWWWWW" subvocally as you picture the pericardium (the thin sac that surrounds your heart) releasing heat, impatience, arrogance, and hastiness.
4. For the rest cycle, repeat the procedure for the liver sound but focus attention on your heart and imagine a bright red

color and the qualities of joy, honor, sincerity, and creativity entering the heart.

5. Do three to six times. For a sore throat, cold sores, swollen gums or tongue, heart disease, heart pains, jumpiness, moodiness, and for detoxifying the heart, repeat nine to thirty-six times.[51]

The fifth healing sound is the *spleen sound*. The associated organs are the pancreas and stomach. The element is the earth, and the season is Indian summer. The negative emotions are worry, sympathy, and pity. The positive emotions are fairness, compassion, centering, and music making. The sound is "WHOOOOOO." The taste is neutral, and the color is yellow.

1. Become aware of the spleen; feel the mouth and spleen connect.
2. Take a deep breath as you place your hands with the index fingers resting at the bottom and slightly to the left of the sternum. Press in with the fingers as you push out with the middle back.
3. Exhale on the sound "WHOOOOO" made subvocally and felt in the vocal cords. Expel the excess heat, wetness and dampness, worry, sympathy, and pity.
4. Breathe into the spleen, pancreas, and stomach. Imagine a bright yellow light and the qualities of fairness, compassion, centering, and music making entering them.
5. Lower the hands slowly to your lap, palms up.
6. Close the eyes, breathe normally, and imagine you are still making the sound. Be aware of sensations and the exchange of energy.
7. Repeat three to six times.
8. Repeat nine to thirty-six times for indigestion, nausea, and diarrhea, and for detoxifying the spleen. This sound, done in conjunction with the others, is more effective and healthier than using antacids. It is the only sound that can be done immediately after eating.[52]

The sixth healing sound is the *triple warmer sound*. The triple warmer refers to the three energy centers of the body. The upper level, which consists of the brain, heart, and lungs, is hot. The middle section, consisting of the liver, kidneys, stomach, pancreas, and spleen, is warm. The lower level, containing the large and small intestines, the bladder, and sexual organs, is cool. The triple warmer sound balances the temperature of the three levels by bringing hot energy down to the lower center and cold energy to the upper center, through the digestive tract. This induces a deep, relaxing sleep. This sound is also very effective for relieving stress.

There is no season, color, or emotion associated with the triple warmer sound.

1. Lie down on your back. Elevate the knees with a pillow if you feel any pain in the small of the back or lumbar area.
2. Close the eyes and take a deep breath, expanding the stomach and chest without straining.
3. Exhale on the sound "HEEEEEEEE," made subvocally, as you picture and feel a large roller pressing out your breath, beginning at the top of the chest and ending at the lower abdomen. Imagine the chest and abdomen are as flat as a sheet of paper, and feel light, bright, and empty. Rest by breathing normally.
4. Repeat three to six times, or more, if you are still wide awake. The triple warmer sound also can be used to relax, without falling asleep, by lying on your side or sitting in a chair.

Try to practice the six healing sounds daily. Any time of the day is fine. It is especially effective at bedtime because it induces a deep, relaxing sleep. Once you have learned the procedure, it only takes ten to fifteen minutes.

Always do the sounds in the proper sequence: lung sound (autumn), kidney sound (winter), liver sound (spring), heart sound (summer), spleen sound (Indian summer), and triple warmer sound.

If you are short on time or very tired, do only the lung and kidney sounds.

The resting period in between each sound is very important. It is the time that you are becoming in touch with, and more aware of, the organs. Often when you rest and smile into the organ, you can feel the exchange of the chi energy in the organ, the hands, and the legs. The head also feels the energy flow. Take as much time as you want during the rest periods.[53]

The Inner Smile

Another ancient Taoist practice is the inner smile. The inner smile directs smiling energy into our vital organs and glands. It is the true smile for all parts of the body, including the organs, glands, and muscles and the nervous system. It will produce a high grade of energy that can heal and eventually be transformed into an even higher grade of energy. I did the inner smile daily while I was pregnant with my girls and both of my labors were very quick and easy. Watch Mantak Chia's video on the inner smile at https://www.youtube.com/watch?v=q2tAXVAP5rA and also https://www.youtube.com/watch?v=oXukcM_b7iM.

Preparation for the Inner Smile

    A. Wait at least an hour after eating to begin.

    B. Choose a quiet spot. It might help in the beginning to turn off your phone. Later on, you will be able to practice almost anywhere with noise, but for now, you need to eliminate distractions in order to develop your inner focus.

    C. Dress warmly enough not to be chilled. Wear loose-fitting clothes and loosen your belt. Remove your glasses and watch.

D. Sit comfortably on your sitting bones at the edge of the chair. The genitals should be unsupported because they are an important energy center. This means men should let the scrotal sac hang free off the edge of the chair. Women should cover their genitals with cloth to ensure no energy is lost through them.

E. The legs should be hips' width apart, and the feet should be solidly on the floor.

F. Sit comfortably erect with your shoulders relaxed and your chin slightly in.

G. Place your hands comfortably on your lap, the right palm on top of the left. You may find it easier for the back and shoulders to raise the level of your hands by placing a pillow under them.

H. Breathe normally. Close your eyes. While concentrating, the breath should be soft, long and smooth. After a while, you can forget about your breath. Attention to the breath will only distract the mind, which must focus on drawing energy to the desired points.

I. Position of the tongue: the tongue is the bridge between the two channels. Its function is to govern and connect the energies of the thymus gland and pituitary gland, and it can balance the left and right brain energies. There are three positions for the tongue. In the beginning, place the tongue where it is most comfortable. If it is uncomfortable to place the tongue on the palate, place it near the teeth.[54]

Smiling Down to the Organs—The Front Line

1. Relax your forehead. Imagine meeting someone you love or seeing a beautiful sight. Feel that smiling energy in your eyes.

2. Allow that smiling energy to flow to the midpoint between your eyebrows. Let it flow into the nose, then the cheeks. Feel it relaxing the facial skin, then going deep inside the face muscles; feel it warming your whole face. Let it

flow into the mouth, and slightly lift up the corners of the mouth. Let it flow into the tongue. Float the tip of the tongue. Put your tongue up to the roof of the mouth and leave it there for the rest of the practice; this connects the two major channels of energy, the Governor and the Functional. Bring the smiling energy to the jaw. Feel the jaw releasing the tension that is commonly held there.

3. Smile into your neck and throat, also common areas of tension. Although the neck is narrow, it is a major thoroughfare for most systems of the body. Air, food, blood, hormones, and signals from the nervous system all travel up and down the neck. When we are stressed, the systems are overworked; the neck is jammed with activity, and we get a stiff neck. Think of your neck as a turtle's neck; let it sink down into its shell and rest from the burden of holding up your head. Smile into your neck and feel the energy opening your throat and melting away the tension.

4. Smile into the front part of your neck where the thyroid and parathyroid glands are. This is the seat of your power to speak. When it is stuck, chi cannot flow. When it is tense and held back, you cannot express yourself. You will be frightened in front of a crowd and cowardly, and communications will break down. Smile down to the thyroid gland and feel the throat open like a flower.

5. Let the energy of the smile flow down to the thymus gland, the seat of love, the seat of fire, the seat of chi, and the seat of healing energy. Smile down into it; feel it start to soften and moisten. Feel it grow bigger, like a bulb, and gradually blossom. Feel the fragrance of warm energy and healing chi flow out and down to the heart.

6. Let the smiling energy flow into your heart, which is the size of a fist and is located a little to the left of the center of the chest. The heart is the seat of love, compassion, honesty, respect, and joy. Feel the heart gradually blossom and send the fragrant warmth of chi love, joy, and compassion

radiating throughout all the organs from the pumping of the heart. Let the smile energy fill your heart with joy. Thank your heart for its constant and essential work in pumping blood to circulate throughout your body. Feel it open and relax as it works more easily.

7. Bring the smile and joyful energy from the heart to the lungs. Smile into every cell of your lungs. Thank your lungs for their wonderful work in supplying oxygen to the body and releasing carbon dioxide. Feel them soften and become spongier and moister. Feel them tingling with energy. Smile into the lungs deep inside and smile your sadness and depression away. Fill the lungs with righteousness that is induced by the love, compassion, and joy from the heart. Let the smile energy of joy, love, and righteousness flow from the heart. Let the smile energy of joy, love, and righteousness flow down to the liver.

8. Smile into your liver, the large organ located mainly on the right side at the bottom of the rib cage. Thank it for its marvelously complex part in digestion—processing, storing, and releasing nutrients—and its work in detoxifying harmful substances. Feel it soften and grow moister. Smile again and get deep into the liver. See any anger and hot temper lying in the liver. Smile it away and let the joyfulness, loveliness, righteousness, and warm chi induce the nature of the liver (kindness) to flow until it is full and overflows out to the kidneys and adrenal glands.

9. Bring the smiling energy into your kidneys, just inside the lower part of your rib cage in the back on either side of the spine. Thank them for their work in filtering the blood, excreting waste products, and maintaining water balance. Feel them grow cooler, fresher, and cleaner. Smile into your adrenals, on top of your kidneys; these produce adrenalin for fight-or-flight situations and several other hormones. Your adrenals may thank you by giving you a little extra shot of energy. Smile again and get deep into

the kidneys. See if there is any fear lying inside the kidneys. Smile with the warmth of joy, love, and kindness and melt your fears away. Let the nature of the kidneys (gentleness) come out and fill them until they overflow to the pancreas and spleen.

10. Smile into your pancreas and spleen. First smile into your pancreas, which is located at the center to the left and above your waist level. Thank it for producing insulin to regulate your blood sugar level and enzymes for digestion. Then smile to the spleen, which is at the bottom and left side of the rib cage. Thank it for producing antibodies against certain diseases. Feel it grow softer and fuller. Smile again into the spleen and pancreas. Feel and see deep inside if there are worries hidden; let the warmth of joy, love, righteousness, kindness, and gentleness melt your worries away. Smile into the virtue of the spleen (fairness). Bring it out and let it grow downward to the bladder and sexual region.

11. Bring the smiling energy down to the genital area in the lower abdomen. For women, this is called the "ovarian palace" and is located about three inches below the navel, midway between the ovaries. Smile into the ovaries, uterus, and vagina. For men, this is called the "sperm palace" and is located one and a half inches above the base of the penis in the area of the prostate gland and seminal vesicles. Smile down to the prostate gland and the testicles. Thank them for making hormones and giving you sexual energy. Let love, joy, kindness, and gentleness flow into the genitals so you can overcome and eliminate uncontrollable sexual desires. Thank your genitals for their work in making you the sex you are. Sexual energy is the basic energy of life.

12. Return to your eyes again. Quickly smile down into all the organs in the front line, checking each one for any remaining tension. Smile into the tension until it is released.[55]

Smiling Down to the Digestive System—The Middle Line

1. Become aware again of the smiling energy in your eyes. Let it flow down to your mouth. Become aware of your tongue and make some saliva by working your mouth and swishing your tongue around. Put the tip of your tongue to the roof of the mouth, tighten the neck muscles, and swallow the saliva hard and quickly, making a gulping sound as you do. With your inner smile, follow the saliva down the esophagus to the stomach, located at the bottom and below the left side of the rib cage. Thank it for its important work in liquefying and digesting your food. Promise your stomach that you will give it good food to digest.

2. Smile into the small intestine: the duodenum, the jejunum, and the ileum, in the middle of the abdomen. It is about seven meters long in an adult. Thank it for absorbing food nutrients to keep you healthy.

3. Smile into the large intestine: the ascending colon, starting at the right side of the hip bone and passing upward to the undersurface of the right lobe of the liver; the transverse colon, which passes downward from the right liver region across the abdomen, the left beneath the lower end of the spleen; the descending colon, which passes downward through the left side of the lumbar region; and the sigmoid colon, which lies within the pelvis, the rectum, and the anus. The large intestine is over one and a half meters long. Thank it for eliminating waste and for making you feel clean, fresh, and open. Smile to it and feel it get warm, nice, clean, comfortable, and calm.

4. Return to your eyes. Quickly smile down the middle line, checking for tension. Smile into the tension until it melts away.[56]

Smiling Down the Spine—The Back Line

1. Bring your attention back to your eyes again.
2. Smile inward with both eyes; collect the power of the smile in the third eye (mideyebrow). With your inner eyesight, direct your smile about three to four inches inside to the pituitary gland and feel the gland blossom. Direct the smile with the eyes into the third ventricle (the power room of the nervous system). Feel the room expand and grow with bright golden light, shining throughout the brain. Smile into the thalamus, from where the truth and power of the smile will generate. Smile into the pineal gland and feel this tiny gland gradually swell and grow like a bulb. Move your smile's eyesight, like a bright, shining light, up to the left side of the brain. Move the inner smiling eyesight back and forth in the left brain and across to the right brain and cerebellum. This will balance the left and right brain and strengthen the nerves.
3. Move the inner smiling eyesight down the midbrain. Feel it expand and soften and go down to the pons and oblongata and to the spinal cord, starting from the cervical vertebra at the base of the skull. Move the inner smiling eyesight, bringing this loving energy down inside each vertebra and the disc below it. Count out each vertebra and disc as you smile down them: seven cervical (neck) vertebrae, twelve thoracic (chest), five lumbar (lower back), the triangular bone called the sacrum, and the coccyx (tailbone). Feel your spinal cord and the back becoming loose and comfortable. Feel the discs softening. Feel your spine expanding and elongating, making you taller.
4. Return to your eyes and quickly smile down the entire back line. Your whole body should feel relaxed. The back line exercise increases the flow of spinal fluid and sedates the nervous system. Smiling into a disc keeps it from hardening and becoming deformed so it cannot properly absorb the

force and weight of the body. Back pain can be prevented or relieved by smiling into the spine.

Smiling Down the Entire Length of Your Body

Start at the eyes again. Direct your inner smile's eyesight. Quickly smile down the front line. Follow the smiling energy down the middle line and then the back line. When you are more experienced, smile down all three lines simultaneously, being aware of the organs and the spine.

Now, feel the energy descend down the entire length of your body, like a waterfall of smiles, joy, and love. Feel your whole body being loved and appreciated.

Collecting the Smiling Energy at the Navel

It is very important to end by storing the smiling energy in the navel. Most ill effects of meditation are caused by excess energy in the head or the heart. The navel area can safely handle the increased energy generated by the inner smile.

To collect the smile's energy, concentrate in your navel area, which is about one and a half inches inside your body. Then, mentally move that energy in an outward spiral around your navel thirty-six times; don't go above the diaphragm or below the pubic bone. Women, start the spiral counterclockwise. Men, start the spiral clockwise. Next, reverse the direction of the spiral and bring it back into the navel, circling it twenty-four times. Use your finger as a guide the first few times. The energy is now safely stored in your navel, available to you whenever you need it and for whatever part of your body needs it. You have now completed the inner smile.[57]

When I was pregnant with my first child, I did the inner smile every day while driving to work. I had an easy, quick, three-hour labor with no complications.

Acupressure has also been used to help women get pregnant. The Hara (CV 6), a special point for toning the abdominal region and enhancing fertility, has been known to help. This point (three finger widths below the belly button) should be used every day for self-treatment (https://www.acupressurewellness.com/ acupressure-point-sea-of-energy-cv6/).

Chapter 3

Reiki

Reiki is one of the more widely known forms of energy healing. Reiki is a healing technique based on the principle that the practitioner can channel energy into the patient by means of touch to activate the natural healing processes of the patient's body and restore physical and emotional well-being. Reiki energy comes from the higher power. The word Reiki is composed of two Japanese words, Rei and Ki. Rei is the higher intelligence or spiritual wisdom that guides the creation and functioning of the universe. Rei wisdom permeates everything, animate and inanimate. Ki is the nonphysical energy that animates all living things. Ki is flowing in everything alive—plants, animals, and humans. The Reiki techniques are known as the Usui System of Natural Healing, after the founder of the system, Dr. Mikao Usui.[58]

Reiki is a technique for stress reduction and relaxation that also promotes healing. Reiki also helps people with emotional distress, pain relief, or any physical, mental, or emotional disorder. It allows everyone to tap into an unlimited supply of that energy to improve health and enhance the quality of life.

Practitioners say that before acting as a channel for Reiki, their physical and spiritual bodies need to be attuned according to ancient and secret symbols revealed to students in three stages over several years. Once the healing channel is opened, it will remain active for life and can be used when required.[59]

A Reiki healing is very simple. You state your intent (what you want the practitioner to treat). Then the practitioner places his or her hands upon or just above the person to be healed with the intent for healing to occur, and then the energy begins flowing. The Reiki energy knows where to go and what to do once it gets there or else is being directed by a higher intelligence. The energy manages its own flow to and within the recipient. It draws through the healer exactly the amount of energy that the recipient needs. All this happens without direct conscious intervention by the healer. The healer's job is to keep the healing space open and to watch and listen for signs of what to do next.[59]

A Reiki treatment feels like a wonderful glowing radiance that flows through you and surrounds you. Reiki treats the whole person, including body, emotions, mind, and spirit, and creates many beneficial effects, including relaxation and feelings of peace, security, and well-being. Many people have reported miraculous results. Reiki is a simple, natural, and safe method of spiritual healing and self-improvement that everyone can use.[60]

Reiki is capable of healing anything because it works at the very fundamental levels of reality. In healing a headache, Reiki may also heal other organs. Reiki also heals on emotional, mental and spiritual levels.[61] The only limits to Reiki are the recipient's willingness to let go of old habits and patterns, to accept change, and to accept healing. At the level where Reiki functions, anything can be changed because all energy is fluidlike and very pliable.

The Reiki ideals are also part of the healing. Their purpose is to help people realize that healing the spirit by consciously deciding to improve oneself is a necessary part of the Reiki healing experience. For the Reiki healing energies to have lasting results, the client must accept responsibility for his or her healing and take an active part in it.

The secret art of inviting happiness
The miraculous medicine of all diseases
Just for today, do not anger
Do not worry and be filled with gratitude
Devote yourself to your work. Be kind to people.
Every morning and evening, join your hands in prayer.
Pray these words to you heart
And chant these words with your mouth.

Usui Reiki Treatment for the improvement of body and mind
—The founder, Usui Mikao[62]

According to an article written by Beth Stapor, PhD, psychologist, licensed professional counselor, Reiki master and teacher with the International Center on Reiki Training, on Reiki and Pregnancy, she knew someone who got pregnant after being given Reiki. Ms. Stapor had a student in her class who had undergone treatment for infertility without success. She had almost given up on having a child. During a weekend where she was taking Reiki I and II classes, she remarked to others in the class that she felt something pop in her lower abdomen. About six weeks after the class, Ms. Stapor received word that she had become pregnant after she returned from her Reiki training weekend. She delivered a healthy baby.[63]

Childless couples came to Hawayo Takota for Reiki. She helped them get pregnant.[64] The International Center for Reiki Training website has stories of people who have been healed of infertility with Reiki. Visit their website at https://www.reiki.org/resources-downloads/reiki-stories?field_story_category_tid=129

Reiki works on the seven chakras of your body.

Chakra Locations

These chakras, the organs they support, mental and emotional issues, and physical dysfunctions are explained in the chart below.[65]

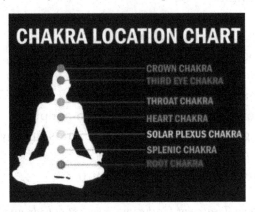

Chakra	Organs	Mental/Emotional Issues	Physical Dysfunctions
First—Root	Physical body support	Physical family and group safety and security	Chronic lower back pain
	Base of spine	Ability to provide for life's necessities	Sciatica
	Legs, bones	Ability to stand up for yourself	Varicose veins
	Feet	Feeling at home	Rectal tumors/cancer
	Rectum	Social and familial law and order	Depression
	Immune system		Immune-related disorders
Second	Sexual organs	Blame and guilt	Chronic lower back pain
	Large intestine	Money and sex	Sciatica
	Lower vertebrae	Power and control	Ob/gyn problems
	Pelvis	Creativity	Pelvic/low back pain
	Appendix	Ethics and honor in relationships	Sexual potency

	Bladder		Urinary problems
	Hip area		
Third	Abdomen	Trust	Arthritis
	Stomach	Fear and intimidation	Gastric or duodenal ulcers
	Upper intestines	Self-esteem, self-confidence, and self-respect	Colon/intestinal problems
	Liver, gallbladder	Care of oneself and others	Pancreatitis, diabetes
	Kidney, pancreas	Responsibility for making decisions	Indigestion, chronic or acute
	Adrenal glands	Sensitivity to criticism	Anorexia or bulimia
	Spleen	Personal honor	Liver dysfunction
	Middle spine		Hepatitis, adrenal dysfunction
Fourth	Heart and circulatory system	Love and hatred	Congestive heart failure
	Lungs	Resentment and bitterness	Myocardial infraction (heart attack)
	Shoulders and arms	Self-centeredness	Mitral valve prolapse
	Ribs/breasts	Loneliness and commitment	Cardiomegaly
	Diaphragm	Forgiveness and compassion	Asthma/allergy
	Thymus gland	Hope and trust	Lung cancer
			Bronchial pneumonia
			Upper back/shoulder pain
			Breast cancer
Fifth	Throat	Choice and strength of will	Raspy throat
	Thyroid	Personal expression	Chronic sore throat

	Trachea	Following one's dream	Mouth ulcers
	Neck vertebrae	Using personal power to create	Gum difficulties
	Mouth	Addiction	Temporomandibular joint problem (TMJ)
	Teeth and gums	Judgment and criticism	Scoliosis
	Esophagus	Faith and knowledge	Laryngitis
	Parathyroid	Capacity to make decisions	Swollen glands
	Hypothalamus		Thyroid problems
Sixth	Brain	Self-evaluation	Brain tumor/ hemorrhage stroke
	Nervous system	Truth	Neurological disturbances
	Eyes, ears	Intellectual abilities	Blindness/deafness
	Nose	Feelings of adequacy	Full spinal difficulties
	Pineal gland	Openness to the ideas of others	Learning disabilities
	Pituitary gland	Ability to learn from experience	Seizures
		Emotional intelligence	
Seventh	Muscular system	Ability to trust life	Energetic disorders
	Skeletal system	Values, ethics, and courage	Mystical depression
	Skin	Humanitarianism	Chronic exhaustion not linked to a physical disorder
		Selflessness	Extreme sensitivities to light, sound, and other environmental factors
		Ability to see the larger pattern	

		Faith and inspiration	
		Spirituality and devotion	

The energy of the first or *root* chakra is tribal power. The word tribal connotates group identity, group force, group willpower, and group belief patterns. The first chakra grounds us. It is our connection to traditional familial beliefs that support the formation of identity and a sense of belonging to a group of people in a geographic location.

The first chakra is the foundation of emotional and mental health. Emotional and psychological stability originate in the family unit and early social environment. Various mental illnesses are generated out of family dysfunctions, including multiple personalities, obsessive-compulsive disorder, depression, and alcoholism.[66]

The second chakra is the *splenic* or *partnership* chakra. Its energy begins to pulsate and become distinct around age seven. With the second chakra, energy shifts from obeying tribal authority to discovering other relationships that satisfy personal physical needs. The second chakra is a powerful force.

This chakra resonates with our need for relationships with other people and our need to control the dynamics of our physical environment. All the attachments by which we maintain control over our external lives, such as authority, other people, or money, are linked through this chakra to our energy field and physical body. The illnesses that originate in this energy are activated by the fear of losing control. Fibroids result from the second chakra creative energy that was not birthed and from life energy that is directed into dead-end jobs or relationships.[67]

Second chakra energy is one of the primary resources we have for coping with the daily events of our lives, providing creative solutions to mental, physical, and spiritual problems or issues. Blocking this energy can lead to impotence, infertility, vaginal infections, endometriosis, and depression.[68]

Men and women both experience energy abortions, which is the aborting of an idea or project. In men and women, energy abortions contribute to physical problems, among them infertility. Many career women who are extremely involved in the birthing of their careers have difficulty becoming pregnant. Some men in the same position also experience prostate problems and difficulty with sexual potency.[69]

Tubal problems and problems with fertility are centered on a woman's inner child, while the tubes themselves are representative of unhealed childhood wounds or unused energy. The flow of eggs can be blocked because a woman's own inner being is not old or nurtured enough, or mature or healed enough, to feel fertile. This energy pattern can cause tubal problems. One part of a woman may remain in prepuberty due to her own unconscious indecision about her readiness to produce life if, on some level, she's not out of the egg herself.[70]

Numerous people who suffer from sexual problems ranging from impotence to infertility to reproductive organ cancer remember having been constantly criticized about their professional skills, ambitions, and accomplishments and their physical appearance. These parents stripped their children of the personal power they needed for health and success.[71]

The third chakra is the *personal power* chakra and becomes dominant during puberty. This energy center contains most issues related to the development of personal power and self-esteem. The third chakra relates to our personal power in relation to the external world.

The third chakra, also known as the *solar plexus*, is the core of the personality and ego. The illnesses that originate here are activated by issues related to self-responsibility, self-esteem, fear of rejection, and oversensitivity to criticism.[72]

The fourth chakra energy is the *heart* chakra, which is *emotional* in nature and helps drive our emotional development. This chakra embodies the spiritual lesson that teaches us how to act out of love and compassion and recognize that the most powerful energy is love.[73]

This chakra focuses on our feelings about our internal world—our emotional response to our own thoughts, ideas, attitudes, and inspirations, as well as the attention we give to our emotional needs.[74]

The fifth chakra is the *throat* chakra. It deals with power of will. This power challenges us to surrender our own willpower and spirits to the will of God. The essence of the fifth chakra is faith.

This chakra lets us progress through the maturation of will: from the tribal perception that everyone and everything around you has authority over you; through the perception that you alone have authority over you; to the final perception, that true authority comes from aligning yourself to God's will.

This chakra represents our emotional perceptions, which determine the quality of our lives more than our mental perceptions. As adults, we are challenged to generate within ourselves an emotional climate and steadiness from which to act consciously and with compassion.[75]

The sixth chakra is the *third eye* chakra. It deals with power of the mind. This chakra involves our mental and reasoning abilities and our skill in evaluating our beliefs and attitudes. It is located in the center of the forehead.

The challenges of the sixth chakra are opening the mind, developing an impersonal mind, retrieving one's power from artificial and false truths; learning to act on internal direction; and discriminating between thoughts motivated by strength and those by fear and illusion.

The sixth chakra links us to our mental body, our intelligence, and psychological characteristics. Our psychological characteristics are a combination of what we know and what we believe to be true, a unique combination of the facts, fears, personal experiences, and memories that are active continually within our mental energy body.[76]

The seventh chakra is our *crown* chakra. It is our connection to our spiritual nature and our capacity to allow our spirituality to become an integral part of our physical lives and guide us. The seventh chakra is directly aligned to seek an intimate relationship with the divine. It is the chakra of prayer. It enables us to gain an intensity of internal awareness through meditation and prayer. It is located at the top of the head.

This chakra contains the energy that generates devotion, inspirational and prophetic thoughts, transcendent ideas, and mystical connections.[77]

Chapter 4

Dahnhak / Body and Brain

I was introduced to Dahnhak through the book *Friendship with God* by Neale Donald Walsch. At the end of the book, he highly recommended the Dahnhak practice for unifying mind and body. There were several centers in my area, so I decided to try it. Dahnhak is a holistic health program to develop our mind and body and enable us to feel and utilize the ki energy, which is the true source of life. It is the modern version of Korea's traditional mind/body training method. *Dahn* means energy, vitality, and origin of life, and *hak* means study, philosophy, and theory.[78] I did Dahnhak two months before I got pregnant with my second child and found it to be very relaxing. They have since changed the name to Body and Brain.

According to the book *Dahnhak: The Way to Perfect Health* by Seung-Heun Lee, the purpose of the practice is to give individuals the opportunity to realize their own personal power. They discover how ki energy, the true source of life, works in their bodies and how they can utilize it for optimal health.[79]

The Body and Brain program is composed of a wide range of forms and movements focusing on yoga, tai chi, meditation, martial arts, and energy healing for all levels. These practices are designed to develop and integrate mind, body, and spirit. The classes are offered at more than one hundred centers throughout the world.[80]

These programs help people lead a healthy life by activating the energy system and maximizing the natural healing power. It also enriches one's emotional life by increasing creativity and sensitivity. Dahnhak / Body and Brain also helps the practitioner make their life significant by awakening them to the truths of life. Through these programs, you will revitalize your body's natural energy through flexibility, strength, and exercises. You will calm your mind and become the master of your thoughts and emotions and discover inner wisdom, deepen your creative power, and let yourself radiate brightness and peace, according to the founder Dr. Lee.[79]

Body and Brain utilizes its own unique five-step energy practice to activate the brain through a deep mind-body connection. First, by developing your capacity to feel energy, you can quiet your mind of cluttered thoughts. You can then experience peace with the flow of life and unleash your innermost wisdom.

From the perspective of energy, all beings in the cosmos exist as one. In the programs, the way to learn about cosmic communication is by breathing. True breathing means taking in the ki energy of the universe and releasing the used, dissipated energy back into the universe. This is known as Dan-Jon breathing.[81]

Don-Jon breathing is a holistic, meditative respiration taking in the cosmic vital energy and accumulate it at a specific point in your body, the lower Dahn-Jon. The lower Dahn-Jon is located two inches below the navel and two inches inside the abdomen. The pure cosmic energy will refresh your mind and body and increase your natural healing power by strengthening the immune system and activating the potential functions of organic mechanisms in your body. This type of breathing will also give you a wider view, a clearer perception, and a higher understanding of yourself and the world.[82]

When practitioners arrive at their goal of a healthy life, they usually extend their intentions toward creating harmonious relationships with their family, friends, acquaintances, and nature. This healthy lifestyle contributes to leading the rest of the world into a new culture supporting happier and healthier human beings.[83]

For more information, the website is www.bodynbrain.com.

Chapter 5

Relaxation Techniques

In this chapter, I will outline several different types of techniques you can use to relax. I have personally used all the methods listed.

Massage

Massage is a great way to recharge your batteries, especially for women who spend a lot of energy taking care of others. Massage fosters a woman's physical, mental and spiritual well-being in a way that few therapies can, says Shawne Bryant, MD, OB, gynecologist, and certified massage therapist in Virginia Beach, Virginia.[84]

Massage may work because it increases circulation. "When you increase the blood supply to the massaged area, you increase the delivery of oxygen and nutrients to the tissues, and you facilitate the removal of waste products," says Dr. Bryant. "In addition, increased circulation promotes healing by increasing the cells involved with fighting infection and disease."[85]

One of the main benefits of massage is the muscles. They may be loosened and relaxed if they are too tight or have knots in them or toned if they are too loose and lack tone. In restoring a balanced tone to the muscles, massage also aids the circulation of blood and movement of lymphatic fluid. Massaging the skin appears to stimulate receptor nerves that transmit a response via the spinal cord to the brain, from where it returns to produce effects in zones of the body supplied by nerves from the same part of the spinal cord. These effects include stimulation and relaxation of voluntary muscles, the opening and closing of blood capillaries, and possibly the sedation of nerve sensors, resulting in pain relief.[86]

Often practitioners recommend massage for women under emotional stress. Infertility is a huge stress for women. Massage definitely helped me deal with the stress of infertility. Infertility affects a person emotionally and mentally. The massage therapist allows people to become aware of tensions they are holding through their touch, and in releasing physical tensions, they can release the worry, anxiety, sadness, or irritability that go with them.

Relaxation Routines

How many times have people told you to just relax and you will get pregnant? I used to get so angry when people told me that. However, we need to know what relaxation really means. Relaxation is not sitting down in front of the television or falling into an exhausted sleep. Relaxation is a state of alert but passive awareness, a state in which our bodies are at rest while our minds are awake. True relaxation is something we may have to rediscover consciously. We must first understand the meaning of stress, its causes and symptoms, and then find ways to change our stressful lifestyle.[87]

Stress is the body's physical, mental, and emotional response to stimuli. Anything that excites, surprises, frightens, angers, or endangers us calls us to adapt or respond. However, modern life presents us with stressful situations continuously and little opportunity to release this stress through action.[88]

Stress affects the hypothalamus, a gland that is very sensitive to emotions, exercise, diet, and light. Because of stress, the hypothalamus may interrupt hormonal messages that lead to ovulation. Stress may cause ovulation to be earlier than usual, or delay ovulation for days or weeks.[89]

In a state of true relaxation, our muscles relax, the heartbeat and breathing slow down, and the metabolism decreases. Therefore, the parasympathetic system is encouraged to regenerate the body's energies. The ability to concentrate without tension is heightened.[88]

A ten-week program for infertile women included training in the relaxation response daily with training in managing stress, exercise, nutrition and group support. Not surprisingly, 34 percent of the women became pregnant within six months of the program. Also, anxiety, depression and fatigue decreased and energy increased.[90]

The Corpse Pose (https://www.youtube.com/watch?v=Mc-38vuwElY)

This is the classic relaxation post practiced in yoga. First, find a quiet place where you will not be disturbed. Wear loose, comfortable clothes, take off your shoes, and undo any belts or buttons. Now lie on you back, feet about eighteen inches apart, palms upward and about six inches from your sides. Allow your legs and feet to roll outward. Check that your body feels symmetrical. Now close your eyes and relax, centering your awareness on the rise and fall of your abdomen.

Tense and Relax Routine

Most people don't realize how tense they are until they truly relax. This routine enables you to feel the contrast between tension and full relaxation.

First, settle yourself in the corpse pose. Now, working up from the feet, first tense, then relax each part of the body—feet, legs, buttocks, stomach, back, chest, shoulders, arms, hands and head. Tense the parts as hard as you can, lifting them a few inches off the floor, and then relax, dropping them down.

Progressive Routine

Lay your hands on your abdomen and breathe in deeply, filling your belly first. Sigh as you breathe out, feeling any tension release with the breath. Repeat a few times, letting go more with each breath out.

Now let your breathing continue at its own pace and depth, and as you breathe out, relax any tension first in the feet. Then, with the next breath out, relax the ankles, then the calves, and so on up the body. Try to really contact each part of the body with your mind and release it completely before moving on. It may help to silently repeat to yourself, "My feet are completely relaxed," and so on, with each breath out, ending with "My whole body is completely relaxed."[91]

Deep relaxation can get your mind off getting pregnant and can help you through the stress of infertility. I used meditation as my relaxation. Every day, I set aside time to just sit in silence and clear my mind. I meditated for twenty to thirty minutes a day.

Stress can affect conception. Two organs that play a major role in the release of stress hormones—the pituitary gland and the hypothalamus, the tiny control center at the base of the brain—orchestrate the reproductive hormones as well.

The normal reproductive cycle depends on a carefully timed sequence of events, orchestrated by hormones released by the brain and the pituitary gland. Stress can disrupt this sequence.

The hypothalamus releases periodic chemical signals that stimulate the pituitary to produce and release luteinizing hormone (LH) and the follicle-stimulating hormone (FSH). FSH stimulates the ovum and the sac of fluid surrounding the follicle to grow to maturity. When the follicle is large and mature enough, the level of the hormone LH rises rapidly, triggering ovulation – the release of the ovum into the fallopian tube.

But when hormones are produced in response to stress, the sequence is disrupted. A variety of stress hormones can disrupt the orderly release of signals from the hypothalamus. The pituitary's secretion of LH and FSH is impaired. As a result, menstruation may become irregular, or ovulation may be suppressed altogether.

Nerve fibers traveling through the spinal cord also link the brain directly to the ovaries, uterus, and fallopian tubes. Through these connections emotional stress may interfere with conception. For example, by disrupting ovulation or the activity of the fallopian tubes may affect your ability to get pregnant. Because of similar links between the brain and reproductive organs, in some men, stress can reduce sex drive and cause impotence. It could lead to retrograde and sham ejaculation, where the sperm is ejaculated backward into the bladder or is not discharged at all, perhaps by changing muscle tone along the male reproductive tract. There is also good evidence from animal studies that severe psychological stress can cause abnormal sperm development, which may impair fertility.[92]

Meditation

To Buddhists, the practice of meditation is essential for the cultivation of wisdom and compassion and for understanding reality. It can help you attain peace of mind and relax. Meditation gives women a chance to turn inward and be kind to themselves. Practicing meditation is like taking a vacation daily. When you nurture yourself, you accrue tremendous benefits. When you meditate regularly, you dramatically reduce your body's response to stress.

Meditation quiets the sympathetic nervous system, slows down the heartbeat and breathing rate, and lowers blood pressure and metabolism. Studies have shown that meditation appears to be most effective in the prevention and treatment of stress-related ailments that have no other basis.

Meditation is a state of heightened mental awareness and inner peace that has mental, physical, and spiritual benefits. During meditation, the brain waves change to a distinctive alpha pattern that resembles deep relaxation and mental alertness. People who meditate regularly can shift into this mode at will, which allows them to deal with stress efficiently and counter certain physical conditions, including high blood pressure and muscle pain.

Ancient traditions believe that we have an inner self that can provide us with wisdom and guidance. Meditation helps us to quiet the mind so we can gain access to this inner source of strength. It also teaches us to control rather than be controlled by our thoughts and emotions. Ordinarily, our minds go from subject to subject with endless associations, which we can detect when we watch ourselves carefully.[93]

By training your attention with meditation, you can increase your awareness of how the internal process begins and decide whether it is useful, and if not, you can stop it or slow it down considerably. Meditation has been said to be doing one thing at a time or living in the present.

Many women tend to live in a state of expectation that prevents them from appreciating the gifts that each moment gives us. We are always waiting for something to happen, and then we will be happy when it happens. It keeps us from being whole. Meditation is a process that returns us to now and allows us to wake up and reevaluate the way we live our lives. Mindfulness meditation is focusing our minds on what is happening around us at this moment.

Practitioners are taught to concentrate on their breathing and its passage through the body as they dismiss any distracting thoughts. Though it sounds simple, mindfulness takes practice, and the longer you practice, the easier the process becomes, according to Daeja Napier, founder of the Insight Meditation Center. "Breathing is the vehicle of transition from our conventional, anxiety-ridden, goal-oriented experience of stressful living into a natural state of functional calm and tranquility."[94]

There are several different types of meditation: mindfulness, journey, vibrational, and movement meditation. Each type is explained below.

Mindfulness meditation works by focusing on your breathing, without using words, images, or sounds, says Napier. "Mindfulness teaches you to work with, rather than against, change in order to establish mental and physical calm."

Settle into awareness. Meditation teachers say it's helpful to begin the day with awareness, even before you get out of bed, Napier says. Use sights, sounds, and senses to tune into your body. Then you're ready to begin meditating.

Find a special place. "Set aside a special place that you can go to each day—a place where you are comfortable and where you're least likely to be interrupted as you meditate," says Napier. "Mark it with something simple like a cushion and a flower. A corner of your bedroom is often a good place to meditate."

Get comfortable. Assume your most comfortable seated position, either on the floor with your back supported or in a chair. You could also lean against a wall, using a cushion for more support.

Just breathe. At first, concentrate on the physical act of breathing, without trying to control or change your normal breathing patterns.

Dismiss distractions. If you get distracted by passing thoughts (and you will, especially in the beginning), avoid following them. Tell yourself that you'll deal with them later. Keep concentrating on breathing (https://www.youtube.com/watch?v=6p_yaNFSYao).

Another type of meditation is journey meditation. Journey meditation combines imagery and visualization to achieve a meditative state. This form of meditation appeals to women who find peace by picturing themselves in a peaceful place, says Eileen F. Oster, licensed occupational therapist from Bayside, New York, and author of *The Healing Mind: Your Guide to the Power of Meditation, Prayer and Reflection*.[94]

Begin by sitting up straight. Get into a comfortable position. Either sit on the floor with your back against a wall or sit in a chair with your feet on the ground and your hands resting on your thighs. Have a pad and pencil nearby. Write down the worries, concerns, or problems that you're afraid will distract you from meditation and promise yourself that you'll deal with them when you're done.

Take a few cleansing breaths. Breathe in slowly and deeply for five counts, then exhale slowly for five counts.

Find a peaceful place. Close your eyes and concentrate on a soothing, tranquil place where you feel safe and calm. As distractions go through your mind, remind yourself that you'll deal with them when you are finished meditating.

A quiet beach is an ideal mental destination for women, says Oster. Picture yourself resting on the sand. Feel the sun on your skin, hear the water lapping the shore, listen for the sounds of seagulls, or see the ships going out to sea. You can use the same routine for any beautiful, serene place that calms you, Oster says.

Do it twice a day. You don't need to spend hours meditating, she says. "Most women will benefit from a 5 to 15-minute meditation practiced several days a week. A good rule of thumb for practicing journey meditation is to do it in the morning and then again later in the day. A peaceful meditative journey as you wake can improve the whole tone of your day," she adds.[95] See https://www.youtube.com/watch?v=6VI4Y87paPs.

Another type of meditation is vibrational meditation. This technique uses the repetition of a word or sound as its focal point. This type of meditation appeals to women who find that making noise is a path to inner quiet, says Oster. "We're taught to be nice and quiet as little girls—ladies aren't loud. Releasing sound and noise helps us release stress," Oster says. So, it's especially helpful to women.

Begin by getting on your feet. Stand with your feet shoulder width apart, your knees slightly bent, and your hips centered, as though you're about to squat. Or you can sit or lie down. Keep your body loose and comfortable with your arms at your sides or on your hips. Begin by taking a few cleansing breaths.

Pick a word, any word. Choose a word that alternates vowels and consonants, like "serenity." The word that you select doesn't have to be a spiritual one, says Oster. It just has to feel good when you say it.

Repeat after yourself. Repeat the word, chant the word, focus on nothing but saying the word over and over again. "Let the sound of the word vibrate through your body. Let the word resonate up from your abdomen and let it go to your hands, and your feet. Let your muscles move as you chant the word," she says.

"Women have a tendency to clench their muscles when they're tense," she observes. "It's important to roll the sound through your body so that you can clear out the tightness in your muscles. Doing so promotes the meditative state of relaxation that feels like a natural high." See https://www.youtube.com/watch?v=k6Xv_yUpvag.

Like yoga, movement meditation combines breathing and gentle, flowing movements to create a meditative state. It appeals to women who tend to achieve a meditative state of mind by moving their bodies, she says.

"Movement meditation allows a woman to draw in *qi* energy from the Earth, which many healers—such as acupuncturists, acupressurists and some massage therapists—regard as the essential life force," says Oster. Qi is energy that moves along meridians, or paths, throughout the body. It is an essential concept in traditional Chinese medicine and other Eastern healing techniques.

"Movement meditation is excellent to do first thing in the morning and can also be a prelude to prayer or another form of meditation," she says.[95]

First, center yourself and concentrate. Take several deep, cleansing breaths. Then move into a relaxed, squatting stance with your knees slightly bent and your hips and pelvis loose. Center yourself by visualizing your feet connected to the soil. Visualize the center of the earth, from which we draw female energy, she says. Concentrate upon and honor the earth.

Focus your awareness. Gently move your body in an undulating, snakelike, swaying motion. See yourself as a flower opening up or as an animal moving though the brush. Dance if you like.

If you want, use sound or music to focus your attention on the movement and on the vibration. Allow yourself to get lost in the sense of movement and the beauty of your body as it moves. Feel the areas of your body that are tight and let the movement loosen them up.[95] See https://www.youtube.com/watch?v=4MLCf9b_OdQ.

The ideal time to meditate is fifteen to thirty minutes a day, preferably at the same time of the day. First thing in the morning is an ideal time.

Imagery and Visualization

Using thoughts to deal with pain, control illness, or reach goals is known as imagery or visualization. Visualization uses the mind to concentrate on visual images, while imagery borrows from all the senses—mainly touch, sound, sight, and smell. To use visualization to relax, you can visualize a restful beach scene. Imagery, however, is more of a self-guided, multimedia event; you imagine hearing the waves, feeling the breeze, and smelling the air.

Guided imagery occurs when someone else shapes the kinds of images that you have, based on what kinds of images seem to have the strongest healing potential for certain conditions. I was fortunate; my meditation teacher also used guided imagery and visualization.

The mind-body connection centers in the hypothalamus, the section of your brain that regulates the autonomic nervous system, which controls automatic processes such as blood pressure. The hypothalamus regulates two branches of the autonomic nervous system—the sympathetic, which responds to stress and gets the heart pumping, and the parasympathetic, which calms the body's responses, explains Judith Green, PhD, professor of psychology and biofeedback in the Department of Behavioral Sciences at Aims Community College in Greely, Colorado, and the author of *The Dynamics of Health and Wellness.*

"These parts of the brain are set up so they'll respond to our thinking and feelings," notes Dr. Green. So, if your brain regulates your body, and your thoughts regulate your brain, it makes sense that you can affect many of your physical responses, including illness.[96]

The relaxation response that visualization and imagery create has a positive effect on the body, notes Howard Hall, PhD, professor, Department of Pediatrics at Case Western University and psychologist at Rainbow Babies and Children's Hospital, both in Cleveland. "Stress causes hormones like adrenaline to flush through the body, which may cause physical symptoms," says Dr. Hall. "Imagery helps counterbalance stress."

Western medicine hasn't always considered the value of mind power in treatment of ailments. Over a two-year period, researchers have performed at least thirty studies involving the use of imagery and visualization. These techniques are most commonly used for everything from headaches to female reproductive disorders, including infertility.[97]

During your visualization, close your eyes, still your mind, and visualize healthy reproductive organs. Visualization exercises can help you manage endometriosis and fibroid symptoms. Visualize your uterus intact, free of unhealthy tissue and growths. Then visualize a baby growing in your healthy uterus. Practice these ten to thirty minutes a day, three to five times a week.

When I was pregnant with my first child, I was concerned about my fibroid. It wasn't in a bad position for the baby, but the doctor said there could still be complications. The hormones of pregnancy could cause the fibroid to grow. So, I said to my fibroid daily, "Whatever purpose you served is over with. I no longer need you in my body. It is time for you to go away." To my amazement, when the doctor performed a sonogram late in my pregnancy, they couldn't find the fibroid! I knew it was gone.

One author says that you can think yourself pregnant. When Boston's Deaconess Hospital introduced a program to help women deal with the stress of infertility, the results were predictable and surprising. Almost all the women who practiced stress-reduction techniques such as yoga, meditation, and breath work felt less stress after finishing the program. Almost 40 percent of them were pregnant six months later. This is not proof that stress causes infertility, but it does suggest that stress contributes to the problem and that stress relief can help solve it, says Alice Domar, PhD, psychologist, founder of the Domar Center for Mind Body and Health, and author of *Conquering Infertility*. She said that fertility drops slightly between age twenty-five and thirty-five, then drops sharply after age thirty-five, and drops dramatically after age forty.[98]

A ten-week program for infertile women included training in the relaxation response with instructions for daily practice and training in stress management, exercise, nutrition, and group support. Results included decreases in anxiety, depression, and fatigue along with increased vigor. Also, 34 percent of the women became pregnant within six months of taking the program.[99]

It is not clear how visualization works, but it encourages activity in the right hemisphere of the brain, which relates to creativity and emotions. Imagery involving sight activates the visual part of the cerebral cortex, sound imagery triggers the auditory cortex, and imagery concerning touch stimulates the sensory cortex.

A vivid image may send a message from the cerebral cortex via the lower brain to the hormonal system and the autonomic nervous system, responsible for body functions such as heart rate and perspiration. Harnessing the power of the imagination may affect these processes and allow the body to find ways of coping with different conditions. If visualization is repeated enough, expectations rise, and the individual begins to act as if the image were a reality. There are two ways of using imagery: active imagery and receptive imagery. Active imagery works with a chosen image to control a symptom or situation or relax the body and mind. Receptive imagery helps patients gain insight into a problem by allowing images to surface that may offer clues to the emotional reasons for certain behavior.[100]

In addition to yoga, meditation, and breath work, the stress reduction program at Deaconess Hospital in Boston teaches women cognitive therapy techniques. This says that you can have better mental and physical health if you get rid of irrational and negative beliefs.

Women with fertility problems often have negative thoughts, telling themselves things like "I'll never be a mother," Dr. Domar says. You can use the following cognitive therapy technique to dispel such notions, she says. The next time you tell yourself that you can't have a baby, ask yourself, "Did the doctor say that I couldn't have a biological child?" The answer is probably no. Then ask yourself, "Is my belief logical?" Again, the answer should be no. By repeating this exercise, you should be able to snap yourself out of illogical, negative thinking.[101] For more information, visit www.domarcenter.com or www.dralicedomar.com.

Another visualization for infertility is called the Fertile Garden. First, state that your intention is to get pregnant. This should be done once a day, for two to three minutes for seven days at the beginning of your ovulation, regardless of how many times you have intercourse. I did this visualization before both of my pregnancies.

To enhance the presence of images, tell yourself to become quiet and relaxed (your intention). Breathe rhythmically, in through the nose and out through the mouth. The exhalations through the mouth should be longer and slower than the inhalations, which are normal, easy, and without effort, not labored or exaggerated. Breathing out longer than breathing in stimulates the vagus nerve, which quiets the body. This nerve originates at the base of the brain and extends down through the neck and sends branches to the lungs, heart, and intestinal tract.

When you are comfortable with your breathing and feel ready to begin your imagery work, instruct yourself to *breathe out three times*. Breathe out, then in; out, then in; then out again—for a total of three out breaths and two in breaths. After this, begin your imagery exercise, breathing regularly.

Close your eyes. Breathe out three times and see yourself going into a beautiful garden. Find a tree and a stream of flowing water. Bathe in the water, allowing it to enter and clean all the ova. Come out and sit under a tree with a lot of sun shining through its leaves. The sky is clear blue. Look up to the right and make a wish or prayer for what you want. Do this quickly. Then call your mate into the garden to join you under the tree. Lie down with him, holding hands. See the blue light forming a dome over you. See what happens with your mate. Afterward, go out of the garden together holding hands, cradling a child between you. Then open your eyes.[102]

The best time to do imagery work is before starting your daily routine. Incorporate it into your waking-up ritual. I did this before both my pregnancies, and it is very powerful!

See https://www.youtube.com/watch?v=dfEllaceRBE.

Polarity Therapy

Polarity therapy is based on the idea that the body has electromagnetic energy patterns that must be in balance. Its creator, Randolf Stone, was a chiropractor, osteopath, and naturopath. His studies included Chinese Medicine, herbology, reflexology, and Ayurvedic medicine, among others. His polarity therapy is a blend of Eastern and Western techniques that concentrate on unblocking the flow of energy in the body.[103] Polarity therapists believe that life energy is kept in constant motion by the pull of opposing poles, which act like magnets. The head and the right side of the body are the positive pole, and the feet and left side are the negative pole. The center of the body, along with the spinal cord, is neutral. Energy flows clockwise between the poles, passing along the central channel, where there are five neutral energy centers of ether, air, fire, water, and earth. The energy centers correspond to the five elements of traditional Chinese medicine.[104] I underwent polarity therapy after my car accident in Hawaii. It made me feel better, and I believe that it was one of the modalities that helped me get pregnant.

Illness and poor health are considered to be the result of stagnation and depletions in the energy currents, and practitioners may use different therapies to restore balance: therapeutic bodywork, nutritional advice, polarity yoga or stretching exercises, and counseling.

For bodywork, touch and manipulation techniques are used to pinpoint and relieve stagnation and encourage the free flow of energy around the body.

Food is believed to contribute to the quantity and quality of this energy. Poor nutrition and digestion may be at the root of many physical problems, and practitioners often prescribe cleansing or detoxifying diets to eliminate harmful products that may have accumulated in the body. A diet containing fresh fruit and vegetables may be recommended.[104]

Polarity yoga exercises, based on the body's natural movements, consist of simple postures designed to help maintain muscle tone, release toxins, and strengthen the spine. Gentle rocking, stretching, and vocal expressions, which will open up the flow of energy, accompany the exercises.

Counseling is used when practitioners feel that negative thoughts are impeding energy flow. They believe that the mind has a direct impact on how the body works. Counseling helps to enhance self-awareness and self-esteem and encourage a positive attitude. Polarity therapy is a blend of Eastern and Western techniques that concentrate on unblocking the flow of energy through the body, says Ruth Kaciak, a bodyworker certified in polarity therapy who works at the Open Center, a wellness facility in New York City.[104]

During a polarity therapy session, the therapist will use a variety of motions (gently applied) aimed at balancing the body's energy. The practitioner usually starts by moving their hands around your head, then down toward your feet, up the body over the five energy centers, finishing back at your head. They will exert different levels of pressure: *neutral,* a light fingertip touch to restore body awareness and balance; *positive,* which aims to stimulate energy by stroking, molding, and rocking the body; and *negative,* which uses sometimes uncomfortable manipulation of body tissue to stimulate the flow of energy. Most people find bodywork relaxing, but in clearing areas of stagnation, it may induce an emotional outburst of anger or grief.

The practitioner also may show you exercises to do at home.[105]

For more information and to find a practitioner in your area, visit the American Polarity Therapy Association at www. polaritytherapy.org.

Yoga

Yoga started as a spiritual discipline six thousand years ago in India and has emerged as a powerful remedy for ailments ranging from menstrual cramps to rashes, and from mood swings to varicose veins, making it a valuable tool for women.

After an hour of yoga, you feel renewed, like you've done an aerobic workout. The result is better posture, increased flexibility, and other benefits, with sweating and jolting your joints and bones.

Yoga is more than just a physical experience; it quiets the mind, so it's very good for relieving stress and improving concentration. Once you finish a yoga routine, you feel very relaxed. Poses that focus on your pelvis help direct energy to the area and ease menstrual problems. Directing energy to the pelvic region may also help with infertility if the energy in that area is stagnant.

The word *yoga* comes from the Sanskrit word meaning "to yoke," joining the mind and body together, says Richard C. Miller, PhD, a yoga instructor and psychologist in San Rafael, California, cofounder of the International Association of Yoga Therapists, and former president and founder of the Marin School of Yoga. "Some people interpret yoga as the union of different forces or energies," he says.[106]

The physical, spiritual, and psychological aspects of yoga make it a useful therapy for health ailments. Physically, yoga can build strength and improve flexibility because it stretches and strengthens the muscles. It's good for the spine because it loosens the back and aids good posture, like correcting slumped, rounded shoulders. This strengthens the body's ability to heal itself. Yoga can also counteract negative emotions such as anger, anxiety, and depression.

"Doing yoga postures and concentrating on breathing is soothing and relaxing. It gives you something else to focus on," says John Orr, an instructor of physical education at Duke University in Durham, North Carolina, and formerly an ordained Theravidin Buddhist monk who practiced in Thailand and India. After people start doing yoga to relieve stress or physical problems, they gradually discover the deeper psychological benefits, says Orr. "In spending quiet time alone, you get to know yourself better. So, yoga keeps you in touch with your physical, mental and spiritual self."[107]

Also, evidence suggests that women who practice yoga are better off emotionally than others. The women who practiced yoga scored much better on tests to measure positive and negative emotions. Poses that focus on your pelvis help direct energy to the area and ease menstrual problems.[108]

To find out more information about yoga, contact the American Yoga Association at www.americanyogaassociation.net or the International Association of Yoga Therapists at www.iayt.org. Many local yoga studios have trial memberships, such as thirty days for thirty dollars. You can also look up yoga classes in your local area. Many different places offer yoga classes.

Chapter 6

Qigong

Qigong is another powerful Chinese healing method. Qigong comes from two words, qi (pronounced chee) and gong. Qi is the universal energy that makes up and flows through everything in the universe. In our bodies, qi means vitality or life force. Gong means to practice, cultivate, or refine, leading to mastery. So, Qigong means to cultivate or refine one's vitality or life force through practice.

As stated earlier, qi energy has two basic forms, yin and yang. For a person to be in perfect health, yin and yang must be in perfect balance. The body has two kinds of qi—internal and external. The qi moving inside the body to keep the body alive is the internal qi. The qi sent out by a healer to help others to heal or do things outside the body is called external qi.

We are all born with qi energy. When qi flows, life continues, and you are healthy. When the flow of qi pauses or is interrupted, you get sick.

Qigong is all about balance—balancing the energy of mind, body, emotions, and spirit. As mentioned before, the Chinese believe that the mind and body are not separate. Qigong can help you to heal physically, emotionally, mentally, and spiritually all at the same time. Through the practice of Qigong, you can experience perfect balance you are meant to have. The benefits of Qigong are numerous.

Qigong combines meditation, focused concentration, breathing techniques, and body movements to activate and cultivate our qi as it flows through the invisible energy channels, the meridians, of the body. It is also based on the same energy meridians as acupuncture.[109]

Qigong enhances the quality of your life by teaching ways to open energy channels and maintain balance in your body. There are four parts to balancing your qi through Qigong: breathing, postures or movement of your body, your mind and meditation, and the sounds.[110]

Wishes, desire, will, imagination, and visualization all come from your mind. They are also all energy and can be very powerful and helpful to you.

In his book *Born a Healer*, Chunyi Lin, creator of Spring Forest Qigong, illustrates how powerful the mind can be in the Finger Growing Game.

Find the lines at the bottom of your palms where your wrists begin. Put these two lines together then put your palms together. Compare the length of your fingers. Most people have fingers that are slightly longer on one hand.

Now, raise the hand with the shorter fingers and put the hand with longer fingers down and lay it gently on your lower stomach. Slightly open the hand that is up. Put a smile on your face, gently close your eyes, and repeat this message in your mind, "My fingers are growing longer, longer, longer, longer ... they are growing longer, longer, longer, and still longer." Say it to yourself with complete confidence. Just know that the fingers on your raised hand are growing longer, longer and longer. Say it for about thirty seconds to a minute and then open your eyes.

After the minute is up, compare your hands again. Your shorter fingers became longer!

Now open your hands. Say in your mind just one time, "My fingers come back to normal." You only need to say it once. Line your palms up at the wrists again, compare your fingers now, and see what has happened. They've gone back to the same length they were when you started.

Put the hand with the longer fingers up in the air and place your other hand on your stomach. This time we want the longer fingers to become shorter. Slightly open the hand with longer fingers and say in your mind, "My fingers are becoming shorter, shorter, shorter …" Focus your mind on those fingers. Feel the energy flowing in the fingers as you say in your mind, "My fingers are becoming shorter, shorter, shorter. My fingers are becoming shorter, shorter, shorter, and even shorter." Again, do this for thirty seconds to a minute.

Find the lines at the end of your palms, put them together, and compare your fingers now. See how longer fingers become shorter?

Now, to put them back to normal, say in your mind, "My fingers go back to normal." Compare your fingers now. They're back to the same length they were when you started.

This is the amazing power of qi and Qigong. The power of your mind influences your qi. Through your focused thought, you sent energy into your fingers, causing the fingers to become longer or shorter. All thoughts are energy.[111]

Here is a simple Qigong exercise to pull energy into your body to attract your goal.

1. Decide on what you want.
2. Get clear of anything in the way of having the goal.
3. Bring energy into your body while holding your intention in mind.

Close your eyes. As you breathe in, imagine the air is energy going to your mental experience. See it travel into your body and to the achievement of your desire. See the energy fueling it. Use your mind while you breathe. In your mind, see your goal. Pretend your energy is magic that will breathe life into your intention.

I practiced Spring Forest Qigong for a half hour every day. It helped me maintain balance between the challenges of working and caring for two children. It calmed me down and forced me to take time out for myself. To learn more, visit www.springforestqigong. com and www.bornahealer.com. You can also look up local Qigong classes in your area. They may have classes at the county or city recreation centers.

Chapter 7

Nutrition

Vitamins and Minerals

The foods we eat play a vital role in our overall health. Because we don't eat like we should, additional vitamins, minerals, and other supplements may be necessary to rebalance our body systems. If fibroids or endometriosis is the problem (I had both), add some bioflavonoids to your diet. They are found in citrus fruits, garlic, onions, and all vegetables. They are plant compounds related to vitamin C. Bioflavonoids seem to reduce excessive bleeding by strengthening capillary walls. They may also lower excessively high estrogen levels. Supplements of 1,000 mg of bioflavonoids daily would be helpful. They are available at health food stores.

Vitamin B helps your liver get rid of excess estrogen, notes Susan Lark, MD, author of *The Estrogen Decision Self-Help Book*. She recommends 50 to 100 mg of vitamin B complex daily. However, when taken over a long period of time, amounts of more than 50 mg of vitamin B_6 can cause unstable gait and numb feet. So, consult your physician first.[112]

Other vitamins and minerals that are essential to fertility include selenium, vitamin C, and vitamin E. Deficiency in selenium leads to reduced sperm count and has been linked to sterility in men and infertility in women. The suggested dosage is 200 to 400 mcg of selenium daily. Vitamin C is important in sperm production. It keeps the sperm from clumping and makes them more motile. Take 2000–6000 mg daily in divided doses. Vitamin E is needed for balanced hormone production. It has been known as the sex vitamin that carries oxygen to the sexual organs. Start with 200 IU daily and gradually increase to 400 then 1000 IU daily.

For men, vitamins and minerals essential to fertility include vitamin B_{12} and zinc. Deficiencies in vitamin B_{12} lead to reduced sperm counts and lowered sperm mobility. Studies suggest that vitamin B_{12} supplementation (1000 mcg daily) can sometimes improve sperm even when there is no deficiency. Zinc is also essential for sperm production, especially when testosterone levels are low. Take 80 mg of zinc daily. Use zine gluconate lozenges or OptiZinc tablets for best absorption. Since zinc lowers copper levels, take 1 mg of copper daily while taking zinc.[113]

Foods

As everyone knows, the type of food you eat affects your body. When I went to a practitioner, she told me that in Chinese medicine, if you were infertile, there was an imbalance of yin and yang. The Chinese believe that infertility is due to insufficient kidney yang. They believe the kidneys affect the reproductive organs. She recommended that I eat the following foods for infertility:

- whole grains, especially barley, a kidney tonic
- cooked vegetables (especially leafy green vegetables like collard greens, kale, mustard greens, broccoli, and cabbage)
- dulse seaweed and kombu seaweed in small amounts (two-tablespoon serving) daily to strengthen kidneys, bladder, and adrenal glands

- beans, especially black beans and adzuki beans, to strengthen the kidneys and adrenals and restore kidney yang
- nuts, especially walnuts and chestnuts
- fish, especially low-fat white fish and salmon, which strengthens kidneys (also bluefish, crab, lobster, caviar, and scallops)[114]
- berries, especially blueberries, blackberries, and black raspberries
- purple grapes
- watermelon
- beets
- pickles
- salty foods, especially tamari and shoyu, miso, *tekka*, and *gamasio*
- tempeh, which has a strengthening effect on kidneys and sex organs when fried and eaten occasionally
- other recommended foods for the kidneys: arame, Irish moss, kelp, nori, wakame, and hijiki

Foods that enhance the water element include barley, adzuki beans, all other beans, buckwheat, and burdock.

My practitioner also told me to eat more warm foods instead of cold foods. Some of these foods I had never heard of, so I had to go to a health food store to find them. Today, you can probably look on Amazon to see if they have them.

To strengthen the outgoing energy and warmth (yang) of a woman's kidneys, use the following herbs in cooking: cloves, fenugreek seeds, fennel seeds, anise seeds, black peppercorns, ginger (dried), and cinnamon bark. Also use walnuts and foods from the onion family (garlic, onions, chives, scallions, and leeks).[115]

Foods to avoid include coffee (especially weakening to the kidneys, adrenals, and sex organs), alcohol (reduces sperm count in men and can prevent implantation of the fertilized egg in women), and high-fat animal foods (especially eggs, pork, and cheese), which block circulation and can cause obstructions in the sex organs. Excessively cold foods shock the stomach, digestion, and kidneys and weaken circulation in the kidneys (kidney fire). Avoid raw foods in the fall and winter when kidneys, bladder, and adrenals are being strengthened. Excess fruit and sugar weaken the kidneys, and soft drinks tax the kidneys. Also avoid drugs and cigarettes. Avoid sugar and reduce earth foods (millet, squash, apples, figs, oranges, tangelos, cantaloupe, bananas, honeydew, raisins, papaya, sweet grapes, tangerines, rutabaga, and artichokes).[116]

When the kidneys are troubled, reduce or eliminate fat and cholesterol foods. Use only small amounts of salt in cooking, avoid salty foods and salt as a condiment, and eat more water foods (watermelon).

Strict adherence to a gluten-free diet has enabled some previously sterile men and women to become pregnant.

Eating a balanced diet is very important to help prepare the body for pregnancy. Do not eat animal fats, fried foods, sugary foods, or junk foods. Eat pumpkin seeds, bee pollen, or royal jelly. Because bee pollen may cause an allergic reaction in some people, start with a small amount and discontinue if a rash, wheezing, discomfort, or other symptoms occur.

Para-aminobenzoic acid (PABA) stimulates the pituitary gland and sometimes restores fertility to some women who cannot conceive.[117]

Eating disorders have also been associated with infertility. In one study, the investigators determined that 16.7 percent of their infertile subjects had eating disorders ranging from bulimia to anorexia. They recommended that a nutritional and eating disorder history be taken in infertility patients, particularly those with menstrual abnormalities. Being very overweight may also hurt your chances to get pregnant.[118]

When you snack, eat healthy snacks. Some of the healthier snacks include Kind bars, Cliff bars, some of the protein bars (check the labels for high sugar content), One, Pirate's Booty, and Kool Foods (www.koolfoods.com).

Chapter 8

Other Modalities

This chapter has a wide variety of general information on different modalities that I have used to get pregnant or just get healthier.

Support Groups

Consider joining an infertility support group for couples or for women and men separately. My husband wasn't interested in joining a couple's group, so I joined a women's group. I found the support group through the local RESOLVE newsletter. I joined the group in September and got pregnant in November. The therapist who led the group told us that many people who join support groups get pregnant shortly thereafter.

The national infertility association RESOLVE is a wonderful organization dedicated to helping infertile couples. They have an extensive library of resources, clearly outlined options, professional services directory, a list of RESOLVE support groups, and current information on the latest assisted reproductive technologies. Visit their website at www.resolve.org.

According to a study at the University of Massachusetts of infertile couples who participated in support groups, thirty of forty-two

(71 percent) achieved pregnancy within six months, compared to twelve of forty-eight couples (25 percent) who did not participate.[119]

It is very helpful to share information with others who have similar fertility problems or groups of people who are all going through the same procedure, such as in vitro fertilization. Sharing information and venting fears in a friendly, supportive atmosphere can reduce the stress of facing the unknown. In addition, sharing practical information on different treatments and physicians can help group members find the approaches that will be most effective for them.

Chiropractic

Chiropractic is a form of alternative medicine mostly concerned with the diagnosis and treatment of mechanical disorders of the musculoskeletal system, especially the spine. Some proponents have claimed that such disorders affect general health via the nervous system, through vertebral subluxation. The main chiropractic treatment technique involves manual therapy, especially spinal manipulation therapy, manipulations of other joints and soft tissues. Its foundation is at odds with mainstream medicine, and chiropractic is sustained by pseudoscientific ideas such as subluxation and "innate intelligence" that reject science. Chiropractors are not medical doctors. A chiropractor is awarded the degree of Doctor of Chiropractic, or DC, after completing at least two years of premedical studies followed by four years of training in an approved chiropractic school. A Doctor of Chiropractic (DC), chiropractor or chiropractic physician, is a medical professional who is trained to diagnose and treat disorders of the musculoskeletal and nervous systems.[120]

According to chiropractic theory, skeletal and joint misalignments caused by accidents, strains, poor posture, and stress are responsible for many types of pain and disease. Any distortion to the spine affects other parts of the body. Chiropractors claim that treatment can ease muscle tension resulting from stress or problems in the internal organs, such as the intestines or uterus. When the skeletal structure functions smoothly, the body's natural healing processes are free to keep the entire system working in harmony. Chiropractic services are used most often to treat neuromusculoskeletal complaints, including but not limited to back pain, neck pain, pain in the joints of the arms or legs, and headaches.[121]

I have been going to a chiropractor for many years and have found it has kept my body healthy because they focus on natural methods and not drugs to keep you healthy. The downside is that it is not fully covered by most insurance companies. If it is, the reimbursement is minimal. Nevertheless, it is worth it for me to keep going because I believe in the way they treat patients.

The aim of chiropractic manipulation is to adjust strains and spinal misalignments on specific joints (also called subluxations) using manual pressure. Sometimes the joints make noises during treatments. The noise is usually caused by nitrogen bubbles inside the joint cavities forming and dispersing in response to the movement.[122] Many others believe that the correction of misalignments increases the potential of the body to heal itself, according to Patricia Brennan, PhD, dean of research at the National College of Chiropractic in Lombard, Illinois.[123]

EFT—Emotional Freedom Technique (EFT) / Tapping

This is another wonderful method that may help you get pregnant. Often, infertility may result from a previous traumatic experience that may be unconsciously preventing you from getting pregnant. Nick Ortner, in his book *The Tapping Solution*, outlines how EFT tapping has helped many people with a wide variety of issues. They have many tapping scripts in the book that you could work with. Also, check out www.thetappingsolution.com for more information.

EFT is a form of psychological acupuncture that uses light tapping with your fingertips instead of inserting needles to stimulate traditional Chinese acupuncture points.[124] The tapping on these designated points on the face and body is combined with verbalizing the identified problem (or target), followed by a general affirmation phrase. Combining these ingredients of the EFT technique balances the energy system and appears to relieve psychological stress and physiological pain. Restoring the balance of the energy system allows the body and mind to resume their natural healing abilities. EFT tapping is safe, easy to apply, and is noninvasive.

Maybe you have some anxiety about changes that will occur when you get pregnant and have a child. There could also be some underlying fears about having a child. Studies have also shown an association between infertility and ambivalence toward pregnancy and children.

I did not use EFT to get pregnant, but I have used tapping for many other reasons and have found it extremely helpful. Other women have used tapping, and it has helped them get pregnant.

Getting started with tapping is easy. There are eight steps in tapping:

1. Choose your most pressing issue and create a reminder phrase.
2. Rate the intensity of your issue on the 0-to-10 scale.
3. Craft a setup statement.
4. Tap on the karate chop point while repeating your setup statement three times.
5. Tap through the eight points in the EFT sequence while saying your reminder phrase out loud. Tap five to seven times at each point.
6. Once you have finished tapping the eight points in the sequence, take a deep breath.
7. Again, rate the intensity of your issue using the 0-to-10 scale to check your progress.
8. Repeat as necessary to get the relief you desire.

The first thing is to focus on the most pressing issue (MPI). What is bothering you the most? It could be something at work, something with your body, family, or something with your spouse. Be as specific as you can and use your intuition. The reminder phrase is a few words that bring to mind the issue. It could be *this fear I feel, this sadness, this frustration, this anger,* and so on.[125]

Now that you know your MPI, give it a number on a 0-to-10 scale. A 10 would be a lot of distress, and a 0 would be none.

The basic setup statement goes like this:

*Even though*_____ (fill in the blank with your MPI), *I deeply and completely love and accept myself.* So, you could say, "Even though I haven't been able to get pregnant, I deeply and completely love and accept myself."[126]

Once you have your setup statement, you can begin tapping. Say it three times while tapping on the karate chop point.[126] The karate chop point is on the outside of the hand. The tapping points are the eyebrow, the side of the eye, under the eye, under the nose, the chin, the collarbone, under the arm and the top of the head.[127] There are several videos on YouTube that walk you through the process: https://www.youtube.com/watch?v=Tj qSyfP2lQ&list=PL9KHqBpZCgA4qxgpOIbQHO9VNzU8tuhRK.

Other General Information

I have included some other general information I found during my research that could be of interest to you.

The ulcer medications Cimetidine (Tagamet) and Ranitidine (Zantac) may decrease sperm count and even produce impotence.

Marijuana and cocaine lower sperm count.

Applying natural progesterone cream may benefit infertile women.

Conception is more likely if the woman is on the bottom during intercourse.

Sperm count reaches its highest level after two or three days of abstinence from sexual activity, but sperm that remains for longer than a month is less effective at fertilizing an egg.

A University of Michigan study showed that intense exercise might result in a drop in the production of hormones involved in potency, fertility, and sex drive.[128]

Also avoid hot tubs and saunas, as they may lead to changes in ovulation and reduced sperm count. However, hot and cold sitz baths are very effective for removing internal congestion and inflammation.

Excessively long showers drain minerals from the body and weaken the kidneys. Loofah brush the body vigorously when showering to promote qi flow.[129]

Antihistamines will dry up cervical mucus along with clearing your sinuses. However, taking Robitussin cough syrup (just Robitussin, not DM, PE, etc.) will help to thin out the cervical mucus in order to make it easier for sperm to pass through.

Ovulation predictor kits are available from drugstores. First Response and Clearblue are some of the most popular test kits. They even have YouTube videos on how to use them. They are based on the fact that the amount of the hormone made by the pituitary gland, the luteinizing hormone (LH), increases greatly approximately twenty-four to thirty-six hours before ovulation. When collecting a urine sample on specific days, the urine is then mixed with a chemical included in the kit, and then urine will change color. This color change indicates that a sudden increase in LH has happened and that ovulation will usually occur within thirty-six hours.

Several studies have indicated that excessive focus on the goal of having a child may result in premature maturation of the eggs in the ovary and subsequent release of eggs that are not ready for fertilization.

Infertility may result from a woman being treated like a dependent child within her marriage. Interestingly, in several studies, the infertile women had resented the onset of their menstrual periods and wanted to remain childlike. They were overprotected by their parents and craved sympathy and affection, and they felt inferior about being female.

The late Niravi Payne, a former therapist in New York City who specialized in infertility, worked with hundreds of infertile women who unsuccessfully tried to achieve pregnancy through medical intervention. She found that many of these women had the psychological characteristics already mentioned and had unconsciously absorbed beliefs about pregnancy, sexuality, and having children that were actually blocking their fertility. For example, some women were actually very unhappy with their current partner but were afraid to say so because they felt they had no alternative but to stay with him. Other women were told by their mothers that having babes could ruin their lives. For those women who were willing to come to terms with unconscious beliefs such as these, Payne reported a subsequent pregnancy rate significantly higher than expected.[130]

Living in artificial light without going outside into the natural sunlight regularly can have adverse consequences on fertility, because light itself is a nutrient. Too many people are stressed at work and don't get outside much. When Dr. Christiane Northrop, ob-gyn, was trying to get pregnant, her basal body temperature rose very slowly at ovulation. Ovulation causes a rise of about 0.8 degrees in body temperature. The ovary produces progesterone at ovulation, which in turn produces a rise in body temperature. She walked outside in the sunlight without glasses or contact lenses for twenty minutes a day. Natural light has to hit the retina in the eye directly. Don't look at the sun directly but be out in the daytime. Within one menstrual cycle, her basil body temperature rose very sharply at ovulation, which was a big improvement in the pattern. She got pregnant within two cycles of doing this, having tried for five months before.[130]

One of Dr. Northrop's patients, after a long bout with endometriosis, surgery, and infertility, healed herself through a process of writing down her feelings and drawing pictures to illustrate them with her left (nondominant) hand. Drawing with the nondominant hand activates the brain's right hemisphere and facilitates getting in touch with imagery and emotions that are important to integrate consciously in the healing process. Memories from childhood often surface as well, because writing and drawing with a hand we don't use usually puts us instantly in a childlike state.[131]

One fascinating study of women undergoing donor insemination noted that after the first few attempts to produce pregnancy, the women, who were previously ovulatory, actually stopped ovulating. The authors concluded that artificial insemination (and any other mechanized, unnatural technique for forcing pregnancy) is on some level a traumatizing procedure that leads to the inhibition of the very process it is trying to accomplish. It cannot substitute for the intimacy and high emotional gratification that occurs naturally when two people come together to create a new life. Interestingly, orgasm has been found to enhance a woman's chances of conception. Involuntary vaginal and uterine movements that promote conception accompany orgasm. Failure to achieve orgasm may lead to circulatory changes in the blood flow to the pelvis, which can affect fertility.[132] Visit her website at www. drnorthrop.com.

Before I became pregnant with my second child, I also did some body wraps. I was trying to lose inches, and body wraps claimed to do just that. They wrap you in bandages soaked in minerals, and you have to keep moving for an hour. Another benefit of these wraps is that they detoxify your body, so you feel better. My last wrap was two to three months before I got pregnant the second time. The wraps may have helped to cleanse my body of toxins to help me get pregnant. For more information on body wraps, visit www.suddenlyslenderinc.com.

Another website to visit is www.dreamsalive.com. It contains valuable information about achieving your dreams and how to live a more fulfilling life by getting what you desire. They have a newsletter that you can sign up for. They outline seven steps to manifesting your desires. They are as follows:

Step 1. Breathe deeply and relax. Close your eyes.
Step 2. State your desire.
Step 3. Visualize success in advance.
Step 4. Feel the core feeling (contentment, fulfillment, etc.).
Step 5. Create a pleasant image (i.e., forest, beach, babbling brook, etc.).
Step 6. Let your desire go and release it to your higher self.
Step 7. Trust that you've done everything you could do.

In his book *The Attractor Factor*, Joe Vitale says that you can write your future. He says just imagine that you already have what you want and write out a scene that describes it. Describe it in such detail that you can feel it! Pretend you are a movie director and write a script for what you want to experience. Really get into it as you write it. Feel it. Sense it. Experience it. He has a notebook full of scripts, and every one he has written has come into reality. He says when you think it and feel it strongly, it comes to be.[133]

Joe Vitale also introduces the concept of yagnas in his book. Yagnas can be performed for any desires, goals, issue, or problems. They can be requested for any purpose or motivation, as long as they are for the highest good.[134] For more information, visit www.yajna.com, www.yagna.by-choice.com, or www.jyotish-yagya.com.

In the book *Ask and It Is Given*, Esther and Jerry Hicks tell people to focus on what they want, not what they don't want. They say most people focus on what they don't want. Where your intentions are focused is what you will receive.[135]

They said there are only three steps to whatever you want to be, do or have. Step 1 – You ask. Step 2 – The answer is given. Step 3 – The answer, which has been given, must be received or allowed.[136]

Also, they say within seventeen seconds of focusing on something, a matching vibration becomes activated. If you stay focused on the thought for sixty-eight seconds, the vibration is powerful enough to begin manifesting that which you say you want.[137] For more information, visit www.Abraham-Hicks.com. They also have many other books, live seminars, and YouTube videos.

Marie Diamond, in her Diamond Feng Shui course, recommends to paint (or buy) a picture of yourself as a mother surrounded by children. She also recommends buying peonies and putting them in your house. For more information, visit https://mariediamond.com. In addition, there are also many more self-improvement courses, books, CDs, DVDs, and trainings at www.learningstrategies.com.

There is even the possibility that you can't get pregnant due to past-life issues that haven't been resolved. I did several sessions with a practitioner on the Akashic records, and he said that several women have gotten pregnant after clearing out past-life issues that they were unaware of.

Spiritual counseling can also be helpful in clearing out blockages and resolving issues. I have had several sessions with a counselor, and it has helped me tremendously.

Another helpful resource is the Release Technique. The release technique is based on the premise that each person has no limits except those that we hold onto subconsciously, and when we let go of our subconscious limitations, we discover that our potential is unlimited for health, happiness, affluence, and materiality. They have live classes, courses, books, CDs, DVDs, and YouTube videos. Visit www.releasetechnique.com for more information.

Energy medicine is also another option. Energy medicine corrects energetic imbalances that are at the foundation of health and vibrancy. In her book *Energy Medicine for Women,* author Donna Eden provides women with a very useful guide to restoring their female health and balance through effective, energy-based therapies.[138] For more information, visit www.innersource.net or www.edenenergymedicine.com. Donna Eden travels around the world healing people of all types of different illnesses and phobias and correcting energy imbalances. She also has many YouTube videos showing energy-enhancing routines. She has several books, CDs, DVDs, and classes on energy medicine. She also has certified practitioners around the world who can help correct energy imbalances.

Notes

Chapter 1: Infertility Facts

1. https://www.reproductivefacts.org/faqs/quick-facts-about-infertility
2. https://www.sart.org/patients/a-patients-guide-to-assisted-reproductive-technology/general-information/assisted-reproductive-technologies/
3. https://americanpregnancy.org/getting-pregnant/what-is-infertlity/
4. https://americanpregnancy.org/infertility/in-vitro-fertilization/
5. The American Fertility Association used to have a website, (www.theafa.org) but it must have been taken down. So I was unable to find where this information came from.
6. https://www.webmd.com/drugs/2/drug-11204/clomid-oral/details/list-sideeffects/
7. Jacob A. Udell, Hong Lu and Donald A. Redelmeier, Canadian Medical Association Journal, CMAJ March 13, 2017 189 (10) E397; DOI: https://doi.org/10.1503.cmaj.160744

Chapter 2: Chinese Medicine

8. Monte, Tom. *The Complete Guide to Natural Healing.* New York, Berkley Publishing, 1997, p. 408
9. Monte, Tom. *The Complete Guide to Natural Healing.* New York, Berkley Publishing, 1997, p. 409
10. Firebrace, Peter, and Sandra Hill. *Acupuncture, How it Works, How it Cures.* Connecticut: Keats Publishing, Inc., 1994, p. 59.

11. Firebrace, Peter, and Sandra Hill. *Acupuncture, How it Works, How it Cures.* Connecticut: Keats Publishing, Inc., 1994, pp 61-66.

12. Firebrace, Peter, and Sandra Hill. *Acupuncture, How it Works, How it Cures.* Connecticut: Keats Publishing, Inc., 1994, p 64.

13. Firebrace, Peter, and Sandra Hill. *Acupuncture, How it Works, How it Cures.* Connecticut: Keats Publishing, Inc., 1994, p 65.

14. Reid, Daniel. *The Complete Book of Chinese Health and Healing.* Massachusetts, Shambhala, 1994, p. 243

15. Reid, Daniel. *The Complete Book of Chinese Health and Healing.* Massachusetts, Shambhala, 1994, p. 244

16. Reid, Daniel. *The Complete Book of Chinese Health and Healing.* Massachusetts, Shambhala, 1994, pp. 160-162

17. Reid, Daniel. *The Complete Book of Chinese Health and Healing.* Massachusetts, Shambhala, 1994, p. 245

18. Reid, Daniel. *The Complete Book of Chinese Health and Healing.* Massachusetts, Shambhala, 1994, p. 246

19. Reid, Daniel. *The Complete Book of Chinese Health and Healing.* Massachusetts, Shambhala, 1994, pp. 246-247

20. Reid, Daniel. *The Complete Book of Chinese Health and Healing.* Massachusetts, Shambhala, 1994, p 248

21. Reid, Daniel. *The Complete Book of Chinese Health and Healing.* Massachusetts, Shambhala, 1994, p 249

22. Reid, Daniel. *The Complete Book of Chinese Health and Healing.* Massachusetts, Shambhala, 1994, pp 250-251

23. Reid, Daniel. *The Complete Book of Chinese Health and Healing.* Massachusetts, Shambhala, 1994, pp 252-255

24. Monte, Tom. *The Complete Guide to Natural Healing.* New York, Berkley Publishing, 1997, p 410

25. Firebrace, Peter, and Sandra Hill. *Acupuncture, How it Works, How it Cures.* Connecticut: Keats Publishing, Inc., 1994, p 51

26. Woodham, Anne and Dr. David Peters. *The Encyclopedia of Healing Therapies.* London, Dorling Kindersley Limited, 1997, pp 90-91

27. Firebrace, Peter, and Sandra Hill. *Acupuncture, How it Works, How it Cures.* Connecticut: Keats Publishing, Inc., 1994, p 32

28. Firebrace, Peter, and Sandra Hill. *Acupuncture, How it Works, How it Cures.* Connecticut: Keats Publishing, Inc., 1994, p 26

29. Firebrace, Peter, and Sandra Hill. *Acupuncture, How it Works, How it Cures.* Connecticut: Keats Publishing, Inc., 1994, pp. 94-96

30. Firebrace, Peter, and Sandra Hill. *Acupuncture, How it Works, How it Cures.* Connecticut: Keats Publishing, Inc., 1994, p 103

31. Firebrace, Peter, and Sandra Hill. *Acupuncture, How it Works, How it Cures.* Connecticut: Keats Publishing, Inc., 1994, p 107

Herbs

32. Woodham, Anne and Dr. David Peters. *The Encyclopedia of Healing Therapies.* London, Dorling Kindersley Limited, 1997, p 267
33. Weil, Andrew MD. *Self-Healing Newsletter.* December 1997
34. Monte, Tom. *The Complete Guide to Natural Healing.* New York: Berkley Publishing, 1997, pp 463-464
35. Elias, Jason, MA Lac, and Shelagh Ryan Masline. *The A to Z Guide to Healing Herbal Remedies.* New York: Wings Books, 1996, p 258
36. Monte, Tom. *The Complete Guide to Natural Healing.* New York: Berkley Publishing, 1997, p 456
37. Gladstar, Rosemary. *Herbal Healing for Women,* New York: Simon and Schuster, 1993, pp 167-168
38. Weed, Susun S. *Herbs for the Childbearing Year,* New York, Ash Tree, 1996, pp 2-3
39. Elias, Jason, MA Lac, and Shelagh Ryan Masline. *The A to Z Guide to Healing Herbal Remedies.* New York: Wings Books, 1996, p 258
40. Balch, James F, MD and Phyllis A. Balch, CNC. *Prescription for Nutritional Healing.* New York, Avery Publishing, 1997, p 515
41. Scott, Julian and Susan Scott. *Natural Medicine for Women.* New York: Avon Books, 1991, pp 130-133

Chi Nei Tsang

42. Chia, Mantak and Maneewan Chia. *Chi Nei Tsang.* New York: Healing Tao Books, 1990, p 1
43. Chia, Mantak and Maneewan Chia. *Chi Nei Tsang.* New York: Healing Tao Books, 1990, p 3
44. Chia, Mantak and Maneewan Chia. *Chi Nei Tsang.* New York: Healing Tao Books, 1990, p 4
45. Chia, Mantak and Maneewan Chia. *Chi Nei Tsang.* New York: Healing Tao Books, 1990, p 318-326

Six Healing Sounds

46. Chia, Mantak. *Taoist Ways to Transform Stress into Vitality.* New York: Healing Tao Books, 1985, p 79

47. Chia, Mantak. *Taoist Ways to Transform Stress into Vitality.* New York: Healing Tao Books, 1985, p 81
48. Chia, Mantak. *Taoist Ways to Transform Stress into Vitality.* New York: Healing Tao Books, 1985, p 81-86
49. Chia, Mantak. *Taoist Ways to Transform Stress into Vitality.* New York: Healing Tao Books, 1985, p 86-90
50. Chia, Mantak. *Taoist Ways to Transform Stress into Vitality.* New York: Healing Tao Books, 1985, p 90-93
51. Chia, Mantak. *Taoist Ways to Transform Stress into Vitality.* New York: Healing Tao Books, 1985, p 94-97
52. Chia, Mantak. *Taoist Ways to Transform Stress into Vitality.* New York: Healing Tao Books, 1985, p 97-100
53. Chia, Mantak. *Taoist Ways to Transform Stress into Vitality.* New York: Healing Tao Books, 1985, p 101-106

Inner Smile

54. Chia, Mantak. *Taoist Ways to Transform Stress into Vitality.* New York: Healing Tao Books, 1985, p 40-42
55. Chia, Mantak. *Taoist Ways to Transform Stress into Vitality.* New York: Healing Tao Books, 1985, p 43-48
56. Chia, Mantak. *Taoist Ways to Transform Stress into Vitality.* New York: Healing Tao Books, 1985, p 48-50
57. Chia, Mantak. *Taoist Ways to Transform Stress into Vitality.* New York: Healing Tao Books, 1985, p 51-55

Chapter 3: Reiki

58. Rand, William Lee. *Reiki, the Healing Touch.* Michigan, Vision Publications, 1991, pp 1-1 and 1-2
59. Woodham, Anne and Dr. David Peters. *The Encyclopedia of Healing Therapies.* London, Dorling Kindersley Limited, 1997, p 107
60. www.reiki.org/faqs/what-is-reiki/
61. Stein, Diane. *Essential Reiki: A Complete Guide to An Ancient Healing Art.* New York: Crown Publishing, 1995, p. 18
62. https://www.reiki.org/articles/original-reiki-ideals
63. https://www.reiki.org/articles/reiki-and-pregnancy
64. Haberly, Helen J. *Reiki: Hawayo Takata's Story.* Maryland: Archedigm Publications, 1990, p 65-66
65. Myss, Caroline, PhD. *Anatomy of the Spirit, the Seven Stages of Power and Healing.* New York, Harmony Books, 1996, pp 97-101

66. Myss, Caroline, PhD. *Anatomy of the Spirit, the Seven Stages of Power and Healing.* New York, Harmony Books, 1996, pp 103-104
67. Myss, Caroline, PhD. *Anatomy of the Spirit, the Seven Stages of Power and Healing.* New York, Harmony Books, 1996, pp 129-130
68. Myss, Caroline, PhD. *Anatomy of the Spirit, the Seven Stages of Power and Healing.* New York, Harmony Books, 1996, p 136
69. Myss, Caroline, PhD. *Anatomy of the Spirit, the Seven Stages of Power and Healing.* New York, Harmony Books, 1996, p 141
70. Myss, Caroline, PhD. *Anatomy of the Spirit, the Seven Stages of Power and Healing.* New York, Harmony Books, 1996, p 144
71. Myss, Caroline, PhD. *Anatomy of the Spirit, the Seven Stages of Power and Healing.* New York, Harmony Books, 1996, pp 150-151
72. Myss, Caroline, PhD. *Anatomy of the Spirit, the Seven Stages of Power and Healing.* New York, Harmony Books, 1996, p 167
73. Myss, Caroline, PhD. *Anatomy of the Spirit, the Seven Stages of Power and Healing.* New York, Harmony Books, 1996, p 196
74. Myss, Caroline, PhD. *Anatomy of the Spirit, the Seven Stages of Power and Healing.* New York, Harmony Books, 1996, p 198
75. Myss, Caroline, PhD. *Anatomy of the Spirit, the Seven Stages of Power and Healing.* New York, Harmony Books, 1996, pp 219-220
76. Myss, Caroline, PhD. *Anatomy of the Spirit, the Seven Stages of Power and Healing.* New York, Harmony Books, 1996, p 237
77. Myss, Caroline, PhD. *Anatomy of the Spirit, the Seven Stages of Power and Healing.* New York, Harmony Books, 1996, p 265

Chapter 4: Dahnhak/BodynBrain

78. Lee, Seung-Heun. *Dahnhak, the Way to Perfect Health.* South Korea, Dahn Publications, 1999, p. 25
79. Lee, Seung-Heun. *Dahnhak, the Way to Perfect Health.* South Korea, Dahn Publications, 1999, p. 27
80. Lee, Seung-Heun. *Dahnhak, the Way to Perfect Health.* South Korea, Dahn Publications, 1999, p. 20
81. Lee, Seung-Heun. *Dahnhak, the Way to Perfect Health.* South Korea, Dahn Publications, 1999, p. 31
82. Lee, Seung-Heun. *Dahnhak, the Way to Perfect Health.* South Korea, Dahn Publications, 1999, pp. 55-56
83. Lee, Seung-Heun. *Dahnhak, the Way to Perfect Health.* South Korea, Dahn Publications, 1999, p. 32

Chapter 5: Relaxation Techniques

84. Loecher, Barbara and Sara Alshul O'Donnell. *New Choices in NATURAL HEALING for Women.* Pennsylvania, Rodale Press, Inc. 1997, p. 214
85. Loecher, Barbara and Sara Alshul O'Donnell. *New Choices in NATURAL HEALING for Women.* Pennsylvania, Rodale Press, Inc. 1997, p. 215
86. Collinge, William MPH, PhD. *The American Holistic Health Association Complete Guide to Alternative Medicine.* New York, Warner Books, 1996, pp. 270-271
87. Stanway, Andrew, MD, MB, MRCP with Richard Grossman, PhD. *Natural Family Doctor - The Comprehensive Self-Help Guide to Health and Natural Medicine.* London, Gaia Books, 1987, p. 60
88. Stanway, Andrew, MD, MB, MRCP with Richard Grossman, PhD. *Natural Family Doctor - The Comprehensive Self-Help Guide to Health and Natural Medicine.* London, Gaia Books, 1987, p. 61
89. Winstein, Merryl. *Your Fertility Signals.* Missouri, Smooth Stone Press, 1991, p. 125
90. Collinge, William MPH, PhD. *The American Holistic Health Association Complete Guide to Alternative Medicine.* New York, Warner Books, 1996, p. 191
91. Stanway, Andrew, MD, MB, MRCP with Richard Grossman, PhD. *Natural Family Doctor - The Comprehensive Self-Help Guide to Health and Natural Medicine.* London, Gaia Books, 1987, p. 63
92. Winstein, Merryl. *Your Fertility Signals.* Missouri, Smooth Stone Press, 1991, pp 94-96
93. Woodham, Anne and Dr. David Peters. *The Encyclopedia of Healing Therapies.* London, Dorling Kindersley Limited, 1997, pp. 174-176
94. Loecher, Barbara and Sara Alshul O'Donnell. *New Choices in NATURAL HEALING for Women.* Pennsylvania, Rodale Press, Inc. 1997, pp 237-238
95. Loecher, Barbara and Sara Alshul O'Donnell. *New Choices in NATURAL HEALING for Women.* Pennsylvania, Rodale Press, Inc. 1997, pp. 239-240
96. Loecher, Barbara and Sara Alshul O'Donnell. *New Choices in NATURAL HEALING for Women.* Pennsylvania, Rodale Press, Inc. 1997, pp. 204-205
97. Loecher, Barbara and Sara Alshul O'Donnell. *New Choices in NATURAL HEALING for Women.* Pennsylvania, Rodale Press, Inc. 1997, pp. 206-207
98. Loecher, Barbara and Sara Alshul O'Donnell. *New Choices in NATURAL HEALING for Women.* Pennsylvania, Rodale Press, Inc. 1997, pp. 464-465
99. Collinge, William MPH, PhD. *The American Holistic Health Association Complete Guide to Alternative Medicine.* New York, Warner Books, 1996, p. 178
100. Woodham, Anne and Dr. David Peters. *The Encyclopedia of Healing Therapies.* London, Dorling Kindersley Limited, 1997, p. 178

101. Loecher, Barbara and Sara Alshul O'Donnell. *New Choices in NATURAL HEALING for Women.* Pennsylvania, Rodale Press, Inc. 1997, pp. 466-467

102. Gerald Epstein, MD. *Healing Visualizations, Creating Health through Imagery.* New York, Bantam Books, 1989, p. 137

103. Loecher, Barbara and Sara Alshul O'Donnell. *New Choices in NATURAL HEALING for Women.* Pennsylvania, Rodale Press, Inc. 1997, pp. 222

104. Woodham, Anne and Dr. David Peters. *The Encyclopedia of Healing Therapies.* London, Dorling Kindersley Limited, 1997, p. 102

105. Woodham, Anne and Dr. David Peters. *The Encyclopedia of Healing Therapies.* London, Dorling Kindersley Limited, 1997, p. 103

106. Loecher, Barbara and Sara Alshul O'Donnell. *New Choices in NATURAL HEALING for Women.* Pennsylvania, Rodale Press, Inc. 1997, p. 309

107. Loecher, Barbara and Sara Alshul O'Donnell. *New Choices in NATURAL HEALING for Women.* Pennsylvania, Rodale Press, Inc. 1997, p. 310

108. Loecher, Barbara and Sara Alshul O'Donnell. *New Choices in NATURAL HEALING for Women.* Pennsylvania, Rodale Press, Inc. 1997, pp. 311, 325

Chapter 6: Qigong

109. Lin, Chunyi with Gary Rebstock. *Born a Healer.* Spring Forest Publishing, New York, 2003, pp. 66-68

110. Lin, Chunyi with Gary Rebstock. *Born a Healer.* Spring Forest Publishing, New York, 2003, p.70

111. Lin, Chunyi with Gary Rebstock. *Born a Healer.* Spring Forest Publishing, New York, 2003, pp.74-75

Chapter 7: Nutrition

112. Loecher, Barbara and Sara Alshul O'Donnell. *New Choices in NATURAL HEALING for Women.* Pennsylvania, Rodale Press, Inc. 1997, p. 464

113. Balch, James F., MD and Phyllis A. Balch, CNC. *Prescription for Nutritional Healing.* New York, Avery Publishing, 1997, p. 514-515

114. Monte, Tom. *The Complete Guide to Natural Healing.* New York, Berkley Publishing, 1997, p. 256

115. My bodywork practitioner, Claire, who I visited when I was trying to get pregnant, gave me these recommended foods to eat to strengthen my kidneys. I don't know where she got them from, but most of them are in reference #114.

116. Monte, Tom. *The Complete Guide to Natural Healing.* New York, Berkley Publishing, 1997, p. 256

117. Balch, James F., MD and Phyllis A. Balch, CNC. *Prescription for Nutritional Healing.* New York, Avery Publishing, 1997, pp. 515-516
118. Northrop, Christiane, MD. *Women's Bodies, Women's Wisdom.* New York, Bantam Books, 1994, pp. 354-355

Chapter 8: Other Modalities

119. I originally got this statistic from the www.resolve.org website when I started writing the book. However, it is no longer on the website.
120. Stanway, Andrew, MD, MB, MRCP with Richard Grossman, PhD. *Natural Family Doctor - The Comprehensive Self-Help Guide to Health and Natural Medicine.* London, Gaia Books, 1987, pp 236-237
121. Loecher, Barbara and Sara Alshul O'Donnell. *New Choices in NATURAL HEALING for Women.* Pennsylvania, Rodale Press, Inc. 1997, pp. 73-74
122. Stanway, Andrew, MD, MB, MRCP with Richard Grossman, PhD. *Natural Family Doctor - The Comprehensive Self-Help Guide to Health and Natural Medicine.* London, Gaia Books, 1987, p 239
123. Loecher, Barbara and Sara Alshul O'Donnell. *New Choices in NATURAL HEALING for Women.* Pennsylvania, Rodale Press, Inc. 1997, p. 74
124. Ortner, Nick. *The Tapping Solution.* California: Hay House Inc, 2013, p. 6
125. Ortner, Nick. *The Tapping Solution.* California: Hay House Inc, 2013, p. 15-16
126. Ortner, Nick. *The Tapping Solution.* California: Hay House Inc, 2013, p. 18-19
127. Ortner, Nick. *The Tapping Solution.* California: Hay House Inc, 2013, p. 21
128. Balch, James F., MD and Phyllis A. Balch, CNC. *Prescription for Nutritional Healing.* New York, Avery Publishing, 1997, p. 516
129. Monte, Tom. *The Complete Guide to Natural Healing.* New York, Berkley Publishing, 1997, p. 257
130. Northrop, Christiane, MD. *Women's Bodies, Women's Wisdom.* New York, Bantam Books, 1994, pp. 353-354
131. Northrop, Christiane, MD. *Women's Bodies, Women's Wisdom.* New York, Bantam Books, 1994, pp. 355-356
132. Northrop, Christiane, MD. *Women's Bodies, Women's Wisdom.* New York, Bantam Books, 1994, pp. 352
133. Vitale, Joe. *The Attractor Factor.* New Jersey, John Wiley & Sons, Inc, 2005, pp 139-141, 126-129
134. Vitale, Joe. *The Attractor Factor.* New Jersey, John Wiley & Sons, Inc, 2005, pp. 123-126

135. Hicks, Esther and Jerry Hicks. *Ask and It Is Given (Learning to Manifest Your Desires)*, California: Hay House Inc, 2004, pp. 26-27, 29

136. Hicks, Esther and Jerry Hicks. *Ask and It Is Given (Learning to Manifest Your Desires)*, California: Hay House Inc, 2004, pp. 47-52

137. Hicks, Esther and Jerry Hicks. *Ask and It Is Given (Learning to Manifest Your Desires)*, California: Hay House Inc, 2004, pp. 109-111

138. Eden, Donna with David Feinstein, PhD. *Energy Medicine for Women.* New York: Penguin Books, 2008, pp. 178-184

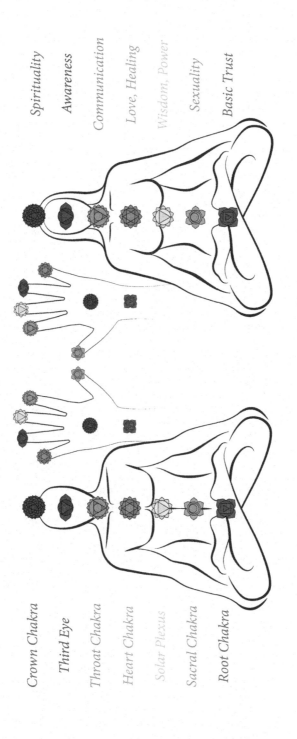

Spirituality

Awareness

Communication

Love, Healing

Wisdom, Power

Sexuality

Basic Trust

Crown Chakra

Third Eye

Throat Chakra

Heart Chakra

Solar Plexus

Sacral Chakra

Root Chakra

List of Index Terms for How to Get Pregnant Naturally

Chapter 3 – Reiki

Chapter 4 – Dahnhak/Body and Brain

Chapter 5 – Relaxation Techniques

Chapter 6 – Qigong

Chapter 7 – Nutrition

Chapter 8 – Other Modalities

Printed in the United States
By Bookmasters